Immunology

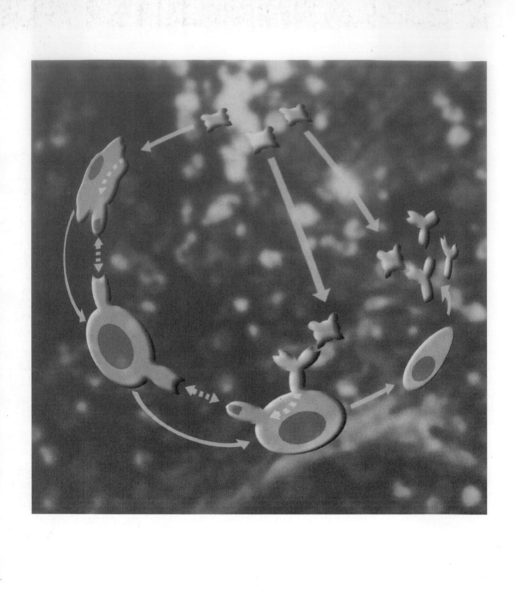

LECTURE NOTES ON

Immunology

GORDON REEVES

MB BS BSc FRCP FRCPath
Professor of Immunology and Head of Department
of Microbiology and Immunology
College of Medicine, Sultan Qaboos University
Muscat, Oman

Visiting Professor in the Immunology of Infection
Imperial College of Science, Technology and Medicine
London

Formerly Professor of Immunology
University Hospital, Queen's Medical Centre
Nottingham

IAN TODD

MA PhD
Senior Lecturer in Immunology
University Hospital, Queen's Medical Centre
Nottingham

Third edition

b

Blackwell
Science

© 1987, 1991, 1996 by
Blackwell Science Ltd
Editorial Offices:
Osney Mead, Oxford OX2 0EL
25 John Street, London WC1N 2BL
23 Ainslie Place, Edinburgh EH3 6AJ
238 Main Street, Cambridge
   Massachusetts 02142, USA
54 University Street, Carlton
   Victoria 3053, Australia

Other Editorial Offices:
Arnette Blackwell SA
   224, Boulevard Saint Germain
   75007 Paris, France

Blackwell Wissenschafts-Verlag GmbH
   Kurfürstendamm 57
   10707 Berlin, Germany

   Zehetnergasse 6
   A-1140 Wien
   Austria

First published 1987
Reprinted 1990
Four Dragons edition 1990
Second edition 1991
Four Dragons edition 1991
Third edition 1996

Set by Excel Typesetters Co., Hong Kong
Printed and bound in Great Britain
at the Alden Press Ltd,
Oxford and Northampton

DISTRIBUTORS

   Marston Book Services Ltd
   PO Box 269
   Abingdon
   Oxon OX14 4YN
   (Orders: Tel: 01235 465500
            Fax: 01235 465555)

USA
   Blackwell Science, Inc.
   238 Main Street
   Cambridge, MA 02142
   (Orders: Tel: 800 215-1000
            617 876-7000
   Fax: 617 492-5263)

Canada
   Copp Clark, Ltd
   2775 Matheson Blvd East
   Mississauga, Ontario
   Canada, L4W 4P7
   (Orders: Tel: 800 263-4374
            905 238-6074)

Australia
   Blackwell Science Pty Ltd
   54 University Street
   Carlton, Victoria 3053
   (Orders: Tel: 03 9347-0300
            Fax: 03 9349-3016)

A catalogue record for this title
is available from the British Library

ISBN 0-632-03812-8 (BSL)
ISBN 0-86542-636-8 (IE)

Library of Congress
Cataloging-in-Publication Data

Reeves, W.G.
   Lecture notes on immunology/
   Gordon Reeves, Ian Todd.
   — 3rd ed.
      p.   cm.
   Includes bibliographical references
   and index.
   ISBN 0-632-03812-8
   1. Immunology. I. Todd, Ian, PhD.
   II. Title.
   [DNLM: 1. Immune System. 2. Immunity.
   3. Immunologic Diseases.
   QW 504 R332L 1996]
   616.07'9—dc20
   DNLM/DLC
   for Library of Congress   95-39681
                                                CIP

Contents

Preface to the Third Edition

This edition is the result of a major revision of the text and graphics with the incorporation of much new material including chapters on immunity and infection and the particular challenge of HIV infection and AIDS. We have also added key or summary points at the end of each chapter and continue to emphasize key words in the text in bold type.

We are particularly concerned about the enormous burden of factual information that the undergraduate student is expected to master and we have limited the dose to what is essential for a clear understanding of the cells, molecules and processes of the immune system and their perturbations in disease. Thus, as previously, we trust that this text will continue to serve the needs of those seeking a straightforward account of immunology whether they are new to the subject or not.

Gordon Reeves
Ian Todd

From the Preface to the First Edition

The undergraduate student meeting immunology during a busy medical or biological sciences curriculum or the qualified doctor attempting to get to grips with the subject for specialist training is often daunted by what appears to be an opaque wall of mystifying jargon surrounding a mass of intricate information. The aim of *Lecture Notes on Immunology* is to provide a concise statement covering the basic facts and concepts that are essential for a first understanding of the subject and its relevance to medicine and allied disciplines. Nomenclature has been simplified and appropriately defined and the major principles introduced in a biological setting. Figures and tables are used to summarize or highlight important information and key words are emphasized in the text in bold type. Brief but carefully selected lists of further reading are presented at the end of each chapter.

This text is based on the teaching modules developed in the Nottingham Medical School which have been designed to provide sufficient grounding to enable students to comprehend and utilize developments in immunology in their practice of medicine. Students often feel more comfortable with the detail when they have glimpsed the whole and for this reason the initial chapter outlines the salient features of immunity culminating in an 'overview of the immune system' presented as Fig. 1.9. Many of these thoughts have been stimulated by the, often penetrating, questions of first-year students as well as the more clinically informed enquiries of medical graduates and I hope that this text will assist the questioning process.

Gordon Reeves

PART I

Immunity and the Immune System

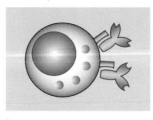

The Nature of Immunity

Infectious diseases, frequently compounded by malnutrition, are still the major cause of illness and death throughout the world. In developed countries, however, the situation has changed dramatically. In Britain, eighteenth century Bills of Mortality listed cholera, diphtheria, smallpox, tetanus and typhoid as major causes of death whereas today the annual mortality statistics emphasize the importance of cardiovascular disease and cancer. The balance has shifted so much that a series of deaths from a particular infectious disease is likely to precipitate the setting up of a committee of enquiry. These changes have been brought about by the introduction of successful immunization programmes in conjunction with chemotherapy and various public health measures. The key role of the immune system in defence against pathogens of many kinds has recently received dramatic emphasis with the rapid spread of the acquired immunodeficiency syndrome (AIDS). Allergic hypersensitivity and autoimmunity are also disturbances of immunity which cause many other kinds of disease, e.g. asthma and glomerulonephritis. Manipulation of the immune system has become of increasing importance in the treatment of disease and in organ transplantation.

This all began with the centuries-old knowledge that an individual who had recovered from a life-threatening infection, e.g. plague, could subsequently nurse another affected individual without fear of contracting the disease again. He or she had become **immune**. The term **immunity** was originally used to indicate exemption from taxes and this meaning still exists in the term 'diplomatic immunity'.

The sequence of events that led to the global eradication of smallpox in 1980 spans more than two centuries and demonstrates vividly the way in which the immune response can be modified to render a previously life-threatening pathogen ineffective in causing disease.

Variolation and vaccination

It is estimated that over 50 million people died of smallpox in eighteenth century Europe. In 1712, a duke's daughter from Nottinghamshire, Lady Mary Pierrepont, eloped with a diplomat, Edward Wortley-Montagu, and later travelled with him when he became British Ambassador to Turkey. She wrote from Constantinople in 1717 concerning the local habit of preventing smallpox by inoculating material obtained from smallpox crusts. She introduced it into England with Royal patronage following initial experiments on condemned criminals and orphaned children. However, this procedure was not without risk of causing smallpox (variola) itself and the high morbidity and mortality associated with it made others look for less dangerous and more effective ways of controlling the disease.

Edward Jenner—a Gloucestershire family doctor—made the important observation that dairymaids, who frequently contracted cowpox (an infection of the hands acquired during milking), were remarkably resistant to smallpox and did not develop the disfigured pock-marked faces of those that had had smallpox infection. Hence the rhyme:

'Where are you going to, my pretty maid?'
'I'm going a-milking, sir', she said.
'What is your fortune, my pretty maid?'
'My face is my fortune, sir', she said.

Edward Jenner had suffered painfully from variolation performed when he was eight years old. The increasing spread of smallpox throughout the population led him to develop the alternative technique of vaccination. This was first performed in 1796 when he inoculated material obtained from cowpox pustules into the arm of a healthy boy. He was subsequently able to inoculate him with smallpox more than 20 times without any untoward effect. This courageous experiment aroused much criticism but Jenner offered his new preventive treatment to all who sought it and performed many of his vaccinations in a thatched hut—which became known as the Temple of Vaccinia—in the grounds of his house at Berkeley. Recently, these buildings have been restored and contain a Jenner Museum and Conference Centre.*

*Further information can be obtained from the Custodian, The Chantry, Church Lane, High Street, Berkeley, Gloucestershire GL13 9BH, UK.

Many other forms of immunization have followed from this work and one of the current goals of the World Health Organization's Tropical Disease Programme is to identify immunological ways of controlling and, hopefully, eliminating other major infections, e.g. malaria (against which vector control has largely failed and chemotherapy is becoming less effective).

Several other kinds of immunological manipulation have proved to be of therapeutic benefit, e.g. the administration of specific antibody in the prevention of rhesus haemolytic disease of the newborn. The advent of monoclonal antibodies of many different specificities offers promise for targeting therapeutic agents to tissues and tumours as well as having many diagnostic applications. Experimental work has shown that the administration of antigen or antibody can be used to turn off specific immune responses—a situation known as immunological tolerance or enhancement. This is of particular relevance to clinical transplantation and the treatment of many immunological and metabolic disorders.

Cardinal features of immune responses (Table 1.1)

An individual who is immune to smallpox will not be protected against diphtheria unless he has also met the *Corynebacterium diphtheriae* on a previous occasion. This illustrates the **specificity** of the immune response. The immune response can detect remarkably small chemical differences between foreign materials, e.g. subtly differing strains of influenza virus, minor substitutions of a benzene ring, or the difference between dextro and laevo isomers. Were it not for the fact that cowpox and smallpox viruses share important antigens, the experiments of Edward Jenner would have been a dismal failure (although he would not have attempted them without the evidence of the milkmaids).

Another feature of immune responses is the **memory** that develops from previous experiences of foreign material—a characteristic which enables immunization to be of clinical value. This altered reactivity may last for the entire lifespan of the individual. The ability of an organism to respond more rapidly and to a greater degree when confronted with the

CARDINAL FEATURES
Specificity
Memory
Self-discrimination

Table 1.1 Cardinal features of immune responses.

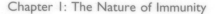

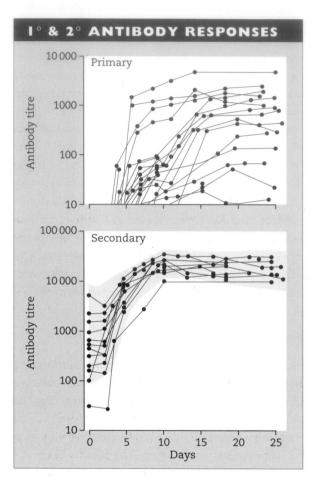

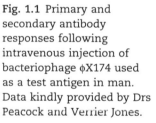

Fig. 1.1 Primary and secondary antibody responses following intravenous injection of bacteriophage φX174 used as a test antigen in man. Data kindly provided by Drs Peacock and Verrier Jones.

same antigen on a second occasion is illustrated in Fig. 1.1. This compares the speed and magnitude of the human response to an antigen which the subjects had not previously encountered (bacteriophage φX174). In the first or **primary** response there is a delay of at least 10 days before the antibody level in the circulation reaches its maximum and this level shows considerable variation between individuals, rarely exceeding a titre* of 1000. In the **secondary** response all individuals respond maximally within 10 days and in all cases the levels attained are of a titre of 10000 or more. As discussed below, the outcome of an acute infection is often a close race between the activities of the replicating pathogen and the adaptive immune response and it is for this reason

*The *titre* is the reciprocal of the weakest dilution of serum at which antibody can still be detected.

that prior exposure, e.g. to a vaccine, can give the host a considerable advantage.

Another important feature of immune responses is **self-discrimination**, which is illustrated in Fig. 1.2. If split-skin grafts are placed on the flanks of rodents, it is possible to observe within 2 weeks whether they have healed well and been accepted (Fig. 1.2a) or whether they have been rejected (Fig. 1.2b). In this experiment, the successful graft was obtained from another animal of identical genetic composition (i.e. another member of the same inbred strain). The rejected graft came from an unrelated member of the same species. These chemical differences are relatively minor and demonstrate not only the recognition ability of the immune system but also the efficient way in which it fails to react against tissue of 'self' origin. Previously, it was thought that components of the immune system failed to recognize self at all but it is now clear that self-recognition does occur in a controlled and regulated manner such that—except in the special circumstance of autoimmune disease—tissue damage does not take place.

BIOLOGICAL RECOGNITION SYSTEMS

Chemical specificity is a feature of various other recognition systems, e.g. enzyme–substrate and nucleotide interactions, although these lack features which characterize immunological responses. It is likely that the recognition component of immune responses has developed from a more basic cellular attribute by which cells are able to recognize each other. Evidence for complementary cell surface interactions has come from several different areas of biological research, e.g. the cellular reaggregation of multicellular invertebrate organisms, e.g. sponges and

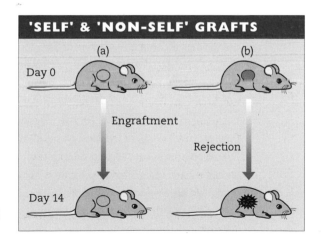

Fig. 1.2 Discrimination between self and non-self illustrated by skin grafting in a rodent. (a) The graft was of 'self' type; (b) the graft was from an unrelated animal.

slime moulds; the processes whereby cells differentially associate during embryogenesis; the way in which synaptic connections are established in the nervous system; and the recognition events involved in pollination and fertilization. Analogy with these other systems suggests that recognition of self is a primary requirement in phylogeny which, in complex mammalian organisms, has developed into a more sophisticated arrangement whereby reactions to self and non-self have been separately harnessed. Antigens and their recognition are discussed in more detail in Chapter 2.

Recognition and defence: a minimal model

Before considering the complexity of the immune system as it exists, it is useful to consider the general design requirements of an immune system in order for it to protect the host organism and display the characteristic features already described. Clearly, the two important biological events are **recognition** of the target pathogen and effective **defence** against it. Using the military analogy, the former is equivalent to reconnaissance and the latter might include artillery support invoked by those in the front line. A major consideration is how many recognition specificities are required and how many kinds of defence, i.e. methods of pathogen destruction, are necessary. The next question to be decided is whether the units that recognize and the units that defend should be combined together or whether a division of labour is preferable in which recognition units and defence units operate as separate entities. These possibilities are exemplified in Figs 1.3 and 1.4, respectively.

Whichever aggressive modality is preferred, it is necessary to plan for rapid adaptation–quantitatively either upwards or downwards–depending on the circumstances. This has implications for the supply of materials and whether the number of recognition and defence units need to be increased in equal proportion. Recognition units, at least, will need to circulate to all parts of the host organism which may be under threat and this will have implications for the size of unit that can permeate into extravascular sites. It is likely that defence units will require greater chemical complexity than those involved in recognition and this has implications for the economy of supplies.

If recognition and defence units occur as separate entities (Fig. 1.4) then a means has to be developed whereby the latter can be specifically recruited to the site where recognition units have detected their target and an arrangement has to be devised for defence units to be activated only when their complementary recognition unit has recognized its

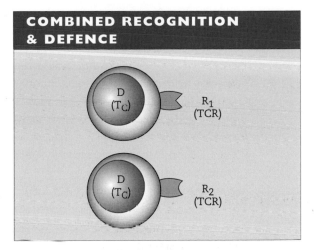

Fig. 1.3 Combined recognition (R) and defence (D) units to deal with a pathogenic invader; R and D units with single recognition specificities exemplified by cytotoxic T cells (T_C). TCR, T cell receptor.

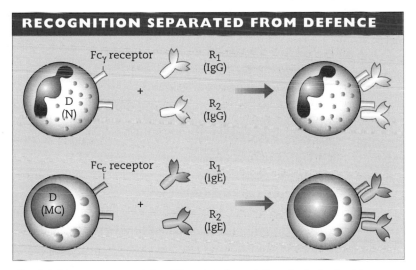

Fig. 1.4 Separate recognition (R) and defence (D) units to deal with a pathogenic invader: R units interact with different D units (e.g. IgG binding to Fc receptors on neutrophils (N) and IgE binding to Fc receptors on mast cells (MC)). R units can have different specificities (R_1, R_2, etc.).

target. Theoretically, the latter could be achieved either by a conformational change developing in the recognition unit (comparable to the steric changes involved in enzyme–substrate interactions) or, alternatively, one could envisage a requirement whereby defence units were only triggered when several of the complementary recognition units become aggregated together on a specific target. It would also be important for the toxic inflammatory products of defence units to be very well contained prior to release or only to be synthesized when the unit has become activated. Furthermore, it might be necessary for inhibitory factors to be present which can limit the scale of the toxic effect of destructive molecules released in proximity to the specific target. If several biologically different kinds of destructive activity are required then different classes of activator will need to be present within the repertoire of recognition units (Fig. 1.4).

As the details of the immune system are reviewed in the succeeding chapters, the reader will realize that each of these different solutions to the basic requirement are found in real life, e.g. cytotoxic T cells are combined recognition and defence units each bearing a single specificity (Fig. 1.3). Immunoglobulins contain a large repertoire of recognition units many of which can activate identical defence units, e.g. complement, but which have also undergone specialization with the development of different classes of activator for different effector systems, e.g. phagocytes vs. mast cells (Fig. 1.4). In summary, the immune system seems to have incorporated most ways of doing things and, as will be seen later, much of its complexity undoubtedly arises from the extensive and varied demands made upon it.

Immunological recognition

The first clue to the identity of immunological recognition units came from studies performed by Paul Ehrlich and his colleagues in the 1890s on factors present in serum which could transfer a state of immunity to a non-immune animal or person. Most of this work focused on toxin-producing organisms, e.g. diphtheria, cholera and tetanus. It was demonstrated that serum factors or 'antitoxins' which developed in the serum of an immune individual were specific for each particular infection. This led Ehrlich to develop his 'side-chain' or receptor hypothesis of immunity in which the numbers of side-chains or receptors available to recognize a foreign specificity could increase in response to an infective stimulus and might possess a separate ability to 'take to itself ferment-like material'. Clearly, he was favouring the possibility outlined in Fig. 1.4. When protein electrophoresis was introduced in the 1930s it was possible to localize these specific serum factors or **antibodies** to the γ-globulin fraction and detailed chemical studies performed by Porter and Edelman culminated in the elucidation of the four-chain structure of these bifunctional **immunoglobulin** molecules in the early 1960s. The structure and function of immunoglobulins are considered in detail in Chapter 6. The plasma cell was identified as the source of serum immunoglobulins in 1948 but their static behaviour and brief lifespan made it unlikely that they were the cells which made first contact with those elements of foreign materials which could generate an antibody response, i.e. **antigens**.

Chase and his colleagues had observed that the immunological reaction induced by the cutaneous application of certain chemicals—known as contact or delayed hypersensitivity—could be transferred from one animal to another by the infusion of lymphoid cells. Gowans took advantage of the natural process whereby **lymphocytes** are separated from the other cells of the blood to form the sole cellular constituent of lymph. He found that animals depleted of lymphocytes by thoracic duct drainage of lymph lost their ability to respond to antigens to which they had previously been immunized and also failed to reject foreign grafts. Immunological responsiveness was restored when their lymphocytes were returned to them by intravenous infusion. It was this work (also in the early 1960s) that caused the lymphocyte to be recognized as the pre-eminent **immunocompetent cell**. However, the link between the freely circulating lymphocyte and the immunoglobulin-producing plasma cell was not established until later.

T AND B LYMPHOCYTES

Peripheral blood lymphocytes are indistinguishable from each other when examined using traditional Leishman or Giemsa stains and it was only when attempts were made to detect the presence of the immunoglobulin recognition units within their surface that a major distinction could be drawn. Using the technique of immunofluorescence it was discovered that about 15 per cent of circulating lymphocytes possess **surface immunoglobulin**. Other work indicated that it was this subset of lymphocytes which transformed into immunoglobulin-secreting plasma cells following contact with specific antigen. Experiments performed in the chicken showed that these lymphocytes required a period of differentiation in a gut-associated lymphoid organ known as the Bursa of Fabricius—and for this reason these cells became designated **B lymphocytes** (Fig. 1.5). The other major subset of lymphocytes responded to antigen independently of antibody, and was found to contain a surface glycoprotein with high affinity for a component of the surface of

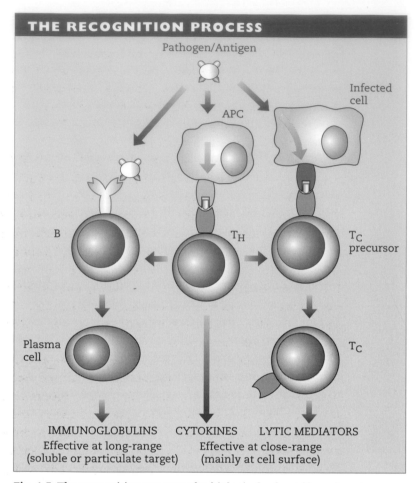

THE RECOGNITION PROCESS

Pathogen/Antigen

Infected cell

APC

B

T_H

T_C precursor

Plasma cell

T_C

IMMUNOGLOBULINS   CYTOKINES   LYTIC MEDIATORS
Effective at long-range   Effective at close-range
(soluble or particulate target)   (mainly at cell surface)

Fig. 1.5 The recognition process: the biological roles of lymphocyte subpopulations. APC, antigen presenting cell; T_H, helper T cell; T_C, cytotoxic T cell; B, B lymphocyte.

sheep red blood cells. The formation of sheep red blood cell 'rosettes' when the two cell types were mixed together provided a useful marker for this lymphocyte subset. It was also demonstrated that these cells required a period of differentiation in the **thymus** and this gave rise to the designation **T lymphocytes** (Fig. 1.5).

The immunoglobulin on the surface of B cells is the specific antigen receptor which, when the B cell transforms into a plasma cell, is secreted as a soluble product capable of interaction with the antigen at a distance from the cell in which it was produced. The antigen receptor on T cells belongs to the same family of surface recognition molecules as immunoglobulins and histocompatibility glycoproteins but it possesses significant differences and recognizes antigen in a different way. Immunoglobulins are designed to interact with pathogens (and parts thereof) which are not intimately associated with cells of the host organism. The T cell receptor, however, is designed so that successful interaction only takes place when antigen is recognized in close association with molecules representative of self cell membranes i.e. the histocompatibility glycoproteins mentioned above. These characteristics are reviewed in Chapters 2 and 3.

Further specialization is evident within both B and T lymphocyte populations, the main subsets of the latter being the helper T cell and the T cells that mediate killer or suppressor activities. The **helper T cell** (**T$_H$**) occupies a central position in immunity, without which the B cell cannot differentiate into the immunoglobulin-secreting plasma cell and without which the **killer** or **cytotoxic T cell** (**T$_C$**) does not become activated from a cytotoxic precursor (T$_{CP}$) (Fig. 1.5). Each of these lymphocyte subpopulations can be identified by various surface markers and although the surface characteristics of suppressor T cells and cytotoxic T cells usually coincide it is still not clear how these two rather different functions are executed.

Most human studies, of necessity, focus on lymphocytes in the circulation rather than in lymphoid tissues but it is in the latter that the large majority of lymphocytes reside (Fig. 1.6). Lymphocytes develop in **primary lymphoid organs**, consisting of bone marrow and thymus, in the adult lymphocytes circulate through **lymph nodes**, the white pulp of the **spleen**, and **mucosa-associated lymphoid tissue** (**MALT**): these locations are referred to as **secondary lymphoid organs**. The total weight of these various lymphoid components can exceed that of the liver. It is at these various sites that the different varieties of lymphocyte come into intimate contact with each other and with specialized antigen-presenting cells. Lymphocytes and lymphoid organs are discussed more fully in Chapters 3 and 4.

Immunological defence

Early observations indicated that additional components, e.g. complement (discovered by Jules Bordet) and phagocytes (first identified by Elie Metchnikoff), were necessary for the successful elimination of pathogens, usually by **lysis** or **digestion**. Different kinds of defence unit do require their own triggering mechanism (as in Fig. 1.4). Figure 1.7 and Table 1.2 show the major defence or effector systems, the recognition units which trigger them and the way they kill pathogens. They have

EFFECTOR SYSTEMS

System	Trigger	Lysis/Digestion
Complement	IgG, IgM, IgA	Extracellular
Neutrophils	IgG, IgA	Intracellular
Macrophages	IgG, IgE	Intracellular
Mast cells	IgE	(Inflammation)*
Eosinophils	IgG, IgE	Extracellular
NK/LGL cells	Lectin†	Extracellular
Cytokines	T cell receptor	Extracellular

* Mast cells do not mediate lysis or digestion, but are a potent source of inflammatory mediators.
† The receptor on large granular lymphocytes (LGL) for targets of natural killer (NK) activity appears to be a carbohydrate binding protein (lectin).

Table 1.2 Effector systems, their triggers and means of lysis or digestion.

THE LYMPHOID SYSTEM

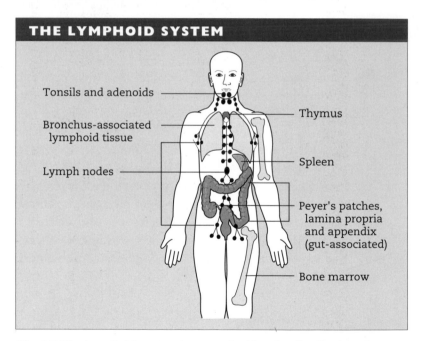

Tonsils and adenoids

Bronchus-associated lymphoid tissue

Lymph nodes

Thymus

Spleen

Peyer's patches, lamina propria and appendix (gut-associated)

Bone marrow

Fig. 1.6 The lymphoid system in man, showing the distribution of primary and secondary lymphoid organs and tissues.

considerable inflammatory and destructive potential and each system has its own internal control mechanisms to reduce the possibility of inappropriate activation and damage to host tissues. The details of these various systems are reviewed in Chapters 7–10. In each case, the terminal act of

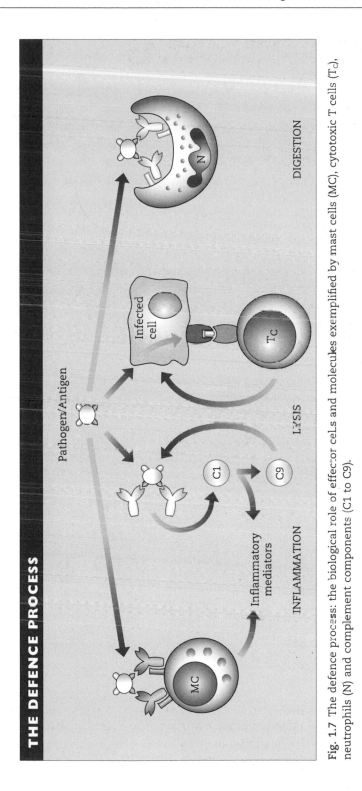

Fig. 1.7 The defence process: the biological role of effector cells and molecules exemplified by mast cells (MC), cytotoxic T cells (T$_C$), neutrophils (N) and complement components (C1 to C9).

THE DEFENCE PROCESS

Pathogen/Antigen

DIGESTION

N

Infected cell

T$_C$

LYSIS

C1

C9

Inflammatory mediators

INFLAMMATION

MC

pathogen destruction is preceded by a series of amplifying events (i.e. **inflammation**) that serves to recruit and harness all the relevant cells and molecules required to achieve the *coup de grâce*, either by intra-cellular digestion or extracellular lysis of the pathogens or infected cells. These amplifying events can be divided into several categories: local **vasodilatation** and increase in vascular **permeability**, **adhesion** of inflammatory cells to the blood vessel wall and their chemical attraction, i.e. **chemotaxis**, **immobilization** of cells at the site of infection, and **activation** of the relevant cells and molecules to liberate their lytic products (Fig. 1.8).

An overview

The complexities of the immune system often seem rather daunting to the novice although students usually find the necessary detail more manageable when they can see how the individual parts fit together into a coherent whole. Figure 1.9 gives a diagrammatic overview of the immune system incorporating the individual components to which

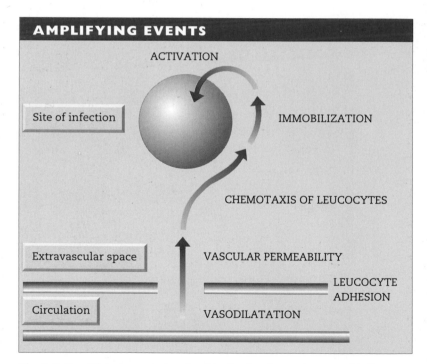

Fig. 1.8 Amplifying events involved in the local recruitment of inflammatory cells and molecules from the circulation into an extravascular site of infection.

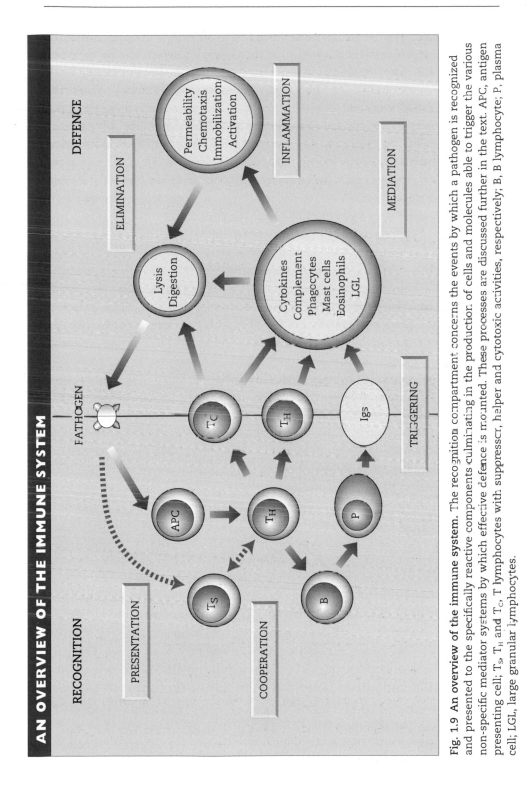

Fig. 1.9 An overview of the immune system. The recognition compartment concerns the events by which a pathogen is recognized and presented to the specifically reactive components culminating in the production of cells and molecules able to trigger the various non-specific mediator systems by which effective defence is mounted. These processes are discussed further in the text. APC, antigen presenting cell; T_S, T_H and T_C, T lymphocytes with suppressor, helper and cytotoxic activities, respectively; B, B lymphocyte; P, plasma cell; LGL, large granular lymphocytes.

reference has already been made and emphasizes the important distinction between those parts of the immune system which specifically recognize the chemical nature of the pathogen and those components which are triggered to act non-specifically and effect its inflammatory destruction. During the recognition process, T and B lymphocytes adapt to the specific antigens to which they are exposed, as in the development of immune memory: this is sometimes termed acquired or **adaptive immunity**. By contrast, the defence mediated by other cell types and complement is termed **innate immunity** since they have a spontaneous capacity for activity regardless of exposure to any particular antigen.

The abundance of means by which recognition and defence can be achieved is surprising and begs the question of why so many alternative pathways have developed during evolution. However, there are similarities as well as differences and the various forms of (a) recognition units, (b) effector systems and (c) lytic processes show considerable homology and may have developed as genetic variants of common ancestral systems.

The stimulus for such diversification arises from the enormous task with which the immune system is confronted, i.e. the constant threat to the survival of the host from a universe of pathogenic organisms ranging from the smallest viruses, through bacteria, protozoa and fungi to metazoan parasites with their often complex life cycles. The remarkable ability of successful parasites to evolve mechanisms by which they can evade the immune response adds a further dimension which is considered in detail in Chapter 11.

Immunopathology

The outcome for the host is often 'survival at a price' and damage to host tissues by the immune system is a common finding during the course of most infectious diseases—a situation referred to as **hypersensitivity** or **allergy**. Furthermore, the development of **autoimmunity** (i.e. immune recognition of self components) is not uncommon during infection and the chronicity of these reactions may be related to the difficulties involved in eliminating certain pathogens from host cells. Some pathogens are also able to initiate various forms of **lymphoproliferative disease** and can cause **immunodeficiency**. **Immunopathology** is comprised of these various deviations from the ideal, many examples of which are found in human disease (Table 1.3). These are described in Part 2 of this text.

IMMUNOPATHOLOGY

Allergy or hypersensitivity
Autoimmunity
Lymphoproliferative disease
Immunodeficiency

Table 1.3 Categories of
immunopathological
disorder.

KEY POINTS

1 Immunity provides protection against pathogenic organisms, and
the functions of the immune system are recognition of these foreign
pathogens and defence of the body against them.
2 Recognition of foreign antigens is a property endowed in T and B
lymphocytes, and immunoglobulin molecules (i.e. antibodies)
produced by the latter. Lymphocytes are thus responsible for the
specificity, memory and self-discrimination of immune responses, as
exemplified in vaccination.
3 Defence is mediated by a range of cells and molecules which
stimulate inflammation and cause digestion or lysis of foreign
pathogens or infected cells.
4 The complexity of the immune system is necessary to deal with the
vast array of pathogenic organisms which can infect the body.
5 Activation of the immune system can also lead to damage to host
tissues and some pathogens can induce abnormal proliferation of the
lymphoid system or cause it to become deficient. These together
constitute the various forms of immunopathology.

Further reading

Ada G.L. (1990) The immunological principles of vaccination. *Lancet*, **335**, 523–526.
Herbert W.J., Wilkinson P.C. & Stott P. (1995) *The Dictionary of Immunology*, 4th edn.
    Academic Press, London.
Mims C.A. (1995) *The Pathogenesis of Infectious Disease*, 4th edn. Academic Press, London.
Nossal G.J.V. (1994) Life, death and the immune system. In *Life, Death and the Immune
    System: Scientific American: A Special Issue*. W.H. Freeman, New York.
Paul W.E. ed. (1993) *Fundamental Immunology*, 3rd edn. Raven Press, New York.
Rains A.J.H. (1974) *Edward Jenner and Vaccination*. Priory Press, London.
Silverstein A.M. (1989) *A History of Immunology*. Academic Press, London.

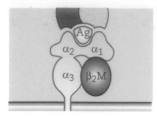

Antigen Recognition

Lymphocytes, as the immunocompetent cells of the immune system, are collectively endowed with the ability to recognize and respond to a wide variety of **antigens**. Most biological materials can serve as antigens, which function either as **immunogens** or **tolerogens** depending on the effect they have on lymphocytes. The recognition and binding of an immunogen by lymphocytes results in the induction of an immune response against the antigenic substance. However, tolerogens induce a specific immunological response of a negative kind, known as **immunological tolerance**, in which an individual becomes specifically unresponsive to subsequent challenge with a normally immunogenic form of the same material.

Factors governing immunogenicity

Whether an antigen induces an immune response or not (i.e. has **immunogenicity**) is dependent on a variety of factors. These are outlined below and listed in Table 2.1.

Nature of the antigen

1 Macromolecular proteins are the most potent immunogens, but polysaccharides, glycoproteins, synthetic polypeptides and synthetic polymers can also be immunogenic. Lipids and nucleic acids are not usually immunogenic unless conjugated to a protein moiety. Nucleoproteins readily induce antibodies reactive with nucleic acids. The more structurally complex a molecule is, the greater is the likelihood of it being immunogenic in most individuals.

2 Smaller molecules are less immunogenic and the smaller the molecule the greater is the variation in response between individuals. The thresh-

IMMUNOGENICITY	
Nature of the antigen	Chemical nature
	Size
	Charge
	Foreignness
Exposure to the antigen	Dose
	Frequency
	Route
	Adjuvants
Nature of the recipient	Age
	Genes
	Nutrition

Table 2.1 Factors governing immunogenicity.

old for immunogenicity varies but is of the order of 1500 daltons molecular weight.

3 Charged residues tend to contribute to the specificity of immunogens as they are usually expressed on the hydrophilic surface of the molecule but uncharged molecules such as dextrans can be immunogenic.

4 The degree of foreignness of a molecule is an important factor. Thus, molecules exhibiting the greatest differences from constituents of the responding animal are usually the most immunogenic, and molecules which do not elicit an immune response in their normal state may do so when denatured. Aggregated molecules tend to be immunogenic whereas aggregate-free proteins administered in soluble form can induce tolerance.

Exposure to the antigen

1 Every antigen has an optimum dose for immunogenicity and in experimental systems doses substantially lower or higher than the optimum can induce 'low zone' tolerance (principally in T cells) or 'high zone' tolerance (in both T and B cells), respectively.

2 Intermittent immunization usually produces a greater response than a period of continuous administration of antigen.

3 The route of immunization is also of importance: oral administration of antigen can induce tolerance to subsequent challenge via the usually immunogenic parenteral route (the Schulzberger–Chase phenomenon).

4 Experimentally, the immune response is usually increased by mixing the antigen with a powerful adjuvant, e.g. a mycobacterial extract, which intensifies the inflammatory response non-specifically.

Nature of the recipient

1 Exposure of very young animals (and of immature lymphocytes generally) to an antigen will often induce tolerance rather than immunity. The immune system also becomes less efficient in the elderly.

2 Significant genetic effects can be observed when relatively 'simple' antigens of modest size are used (e.g. insulin). Thus, animals of a single species, but possessing different relevant genes, may differ in their ability to respond to such antigens. This variation has been shown to associate with particular phenotypes of both the HLA and immunoglobulin allotype systems (see p. 33 & 83).

3 Malnutrition or metabolic disturbances (as in uncontrolled diabetes) impair immune responsiveness.

RECEPTOR–ANTIGEN INTERACTIONS

B and T lymphocytes possess different surface receptors for antigens, and immunoglobulins or antibodies are a secreted form of the receptors expressed by B cells. The part of an antigen recognized by the **antigen combining sites** of these receptors is called an **antigenic determinant** or **epitope**, and usually consists of a small portion of the foreign material (Fig. 2.1). Studies using defined antigens have indicated that the size of an antigenic determinant recognized by an antibody's combining site is roughly equivalent to a tetrapeptide or hexasaccharide. Thus, even some of the simplest viruses or bacterial toxins possess numerous potential determinants.

The binding of an antigenic determinant to a receptor combining site is analogous to hormone—receptor or substrate—enzyme interactions in being dependent on non-covalent intermolecular attractive forces. Both electrostatic interactions (ionic, hydrogen bonding and Van der Waal's forces) and hydrophobic interactions contribute to this binding. These can only occur if the epitope and combining site come into very close contact. Strong association is therefore dependent on a close fit between the determinant and combining site to maximize the opportunities for attractive interactions between complementary chemical groups in appropriate positions. Thus, an antibody, for example, shows **specificity** for an epitope whose shape and charge properties are complementary to those of its own combining site, so that they bind together with a high **affinity**. The same antibody lacks specificity for an antigenic determinant with a very different shape and/or charge for which its binding affinity is negligible. If, however, they are sufficiently complementary to show a degree of interaction, then the antibody is said to **cross-react** with this other determinant (Fig. 2.2).

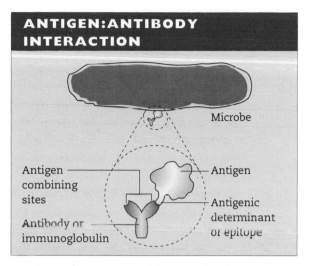

Fig. 2.1 The interaction between an antibody and an antigen.

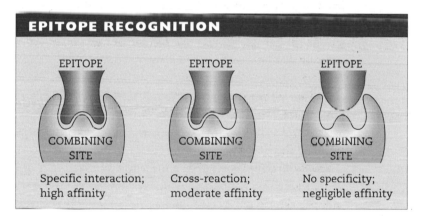

Fig. 2.2 The interaction between an antigen combining site and epitopes of different shapes.

Antigen receptors of B and T lymphocytes

The first antigen-specific recognition units of the immune system to be identified were the immunoglobulins. These are secreted by plasma cells derived from activated B cells. The polypeptide chains of immunoglobulins are made up of a series of disulphide-bonded peptide loops of β-pleated sheets called **domains**, which are composed of sequences of about 110 amino acids. A number of protein molecules expressed on the surface of lymphocytes and other cells involved in immune responses contain domains which show considerable similarity in amino acid sequence and three-dimensional structure to immunoglobulin domains. These molecules constitute the **immunoglobulin super-family**, and some of them are illustrated in Fig. 2.3.

B lymphocytes express immunoglobulin molecules in their surface membranes and these can be detected by immunofluorescence (see Chapters 4 and 6). Surface immunoglobulins are the B cell receptors for antigen (Figs 2.3 and 2.4), and differ in structure from secreted immunoglobulins (described in Chapter 6) in having a carboxyterminal amino acid sequence which anchors them in the cell membrane. A receptor is made up of two identical heavy chains (molecular weight between 50 000 and 70 000 daltons each) and two identical light chains (molecular weight 25 000 daltons). It has a pair of identical binding sites for antigen, each composed of the **variable** (V) domains of one heavy and one light chain (Fig. 2.4) which vary in amino acid sequence among the large variety of receptors with different antigenic specificities. The **constant** (C) domains do not contribute directly to antigen recognition and differ within heavy chains only between the five **classes** of immunoglobulins (IgM, IgD, IgG, IgA and IgE), and differ within light chains between the two types, called κ and λ, both of which can associate with the five types of heavy chains.

The T cell receptor for antigen is a member of the immunoglobulin superfamily (Fig. 2.3) and consists of two polypeptide chains (α and β) which form a disulphide-linked dimer. The α and β chains each have one constant domain proximal to the cell membrane and one variable domain. The two variable domains form the single combining site of the receptor distal to the cell membrane (Fig. 2.4). A minority of T cells express an alternative form of receptor composed of γ and δ chains, instead of α and β chains. The overall structure of the γδ-dimer is similar to the αβ receptor, containing two constant and two variable domains. Although the role of γδ-expressing T cells has yet to be clarified, they accumulate in the epidermis and intestinal epithelium and may be important in the response to infection.

All the antigen receptors expressed by a single B or T cell have identical combining sites so that each lymphocyte has a particular antigenic specificity. The individual, however, possesses about 10^8 varieties of lymphocyte receptor and it is this diversity of receptors which endows the immune system with the potential to respond to a vast array of antigens, any of which may gain entry to the body. The genetic mechanisms underlying the generation of this diversity are described in Chapter 6.

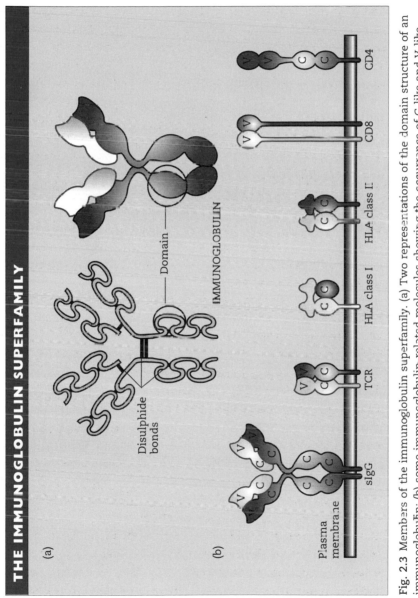

Fig. 2.3 Members of the immunoglobulin superfamily. (a) Two representations of the domain structure of an immunoglobulin; (b) some immunoglobulin-related molecules showing the occurrence of C-like and V-like domains (although the V-like domains in CD4 and CD8 are not actually variable).

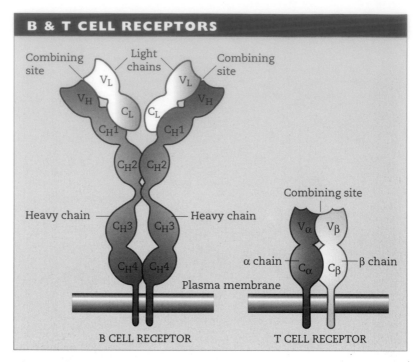

Fig. 2.4 The structure of B and T cell receptors for antigen (the former exemplified by monomeric IgM).

The proliferation of a lymphocyte will result in a **clone** of cells with receptors of identical specificity. From the repertoire of specificities available, an antigen will selectively interact with those clones of lymphocytes whose receptors bind it with highest affinity, resulting in their activation and proliferation. It is this **clonal selection** which ensures that an immune response is specific for the immunizing antigen (Fig. 2.5).

Antigen recognition by B and T lymphocytes

The form in which antigen is recognized and bound by receptors on B and T lymphocytes is very different (Fig. 2.6). This reflects the different functions of B and T cells following activation by antigen.

An activated B cell can mature into a plasma cell which secretes large numbers of antibody molecules with the same antigenic specificity as the receptors of the B cell from which it arose (Fig. 2.6). The function of antibody molecules is to bind directly to the stimulating antigen (which

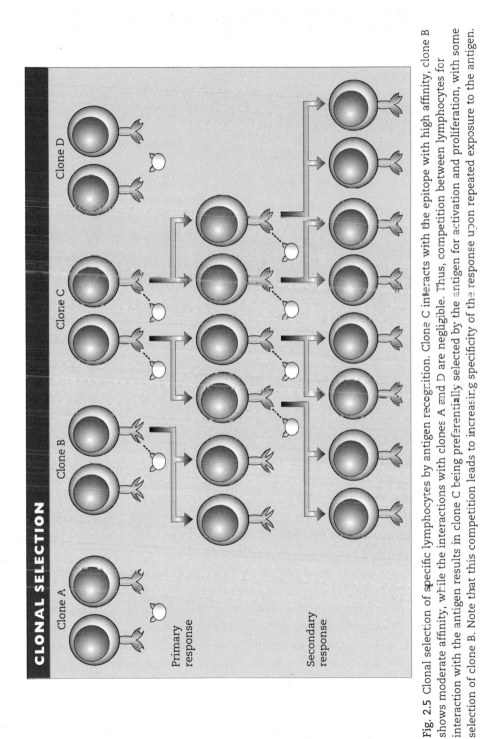

Fig. 2.5 Clonal selection of specific lymphocytes by antigen recognition. Clone C interacts with the epitope with high affinity, clone B shows moderate affinity, while the interactions with clones A and D are negligible. Thus, competition between lymphocytes for interaction with the antigen results in clone C being preferentially selected by the antigen for activation and proliferation, with some selection of clone B. Note that this competition leads to increasing specificity of the response upon repeated exposure to the antigen.

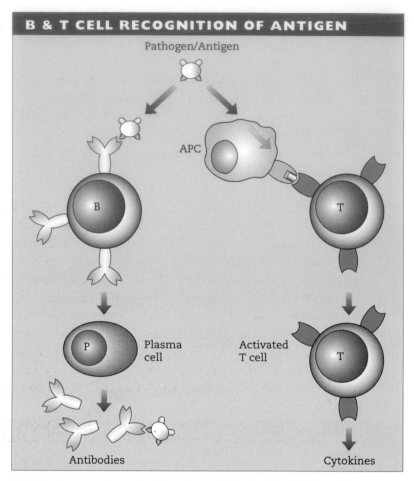

Fig. 2.6 A comparison of antigen recognition by B and T lymphocytes. APC, antigen presenting cell.

may, for example, be a bacterium or a virus) and thereby either neutralize its activity or trigger immune defence mechanisms which bring about its elimination. In practice this means that a B cell antigen receptor or an antibody can interact with an antigen in its native, unmodified state, e.g. on the surface of a bacterium or in free solution (Fig. 2.6). It is thus not surprising that epitopes recognized by B cells and antibodies are often the most accessible regions on the surface of antigen molecules.

T cells either regulate the activity of other immune cells, or they kill infected cells. Thus, T cells are required to interact with other cell types to achieve their functional effects. This may explain why, in contrast to B cells, T cells can only recognize, and be activated by, antigen bound to specialized cell surface glycoproteins (called **HLA molecules** in humans) encoded by genes of the major histocompatibility complex (see below). Cells bearing surface antigen bound to HLA molecules are termed **antigen presenting cells** if their role is to activate T cells (Fig. 2.6), or **target cells** if they are killed by T cells.

T cell receptors do not bind antigen or HLA molecules alone, and only bind effectively to a combination of both. This is called **associative** or **dual recognition**. Most unmodified antigens are unable to associate effectively with HLA molecules, but can do so when they have been processed by the antigen presenting cell. **Antigen processing** involves partial degradation by enzymes to yield peptides, some of which are of the appropriate length and amino acid sequence to bind to HLA molecules and hence can serve as T cell epitopes (see pp. 51–52). These antigenic determinants can be derived from any part of the original antigen and thus, unlike the B cell epitopes discussed above, may not be exposed on the surface of the antigen in its native configuration. A corollary of this is that B and T cells may interact with totally different epitopes yet still show specificity for the same overall antigen. This is illustrated in Fig. 2.7 using as an example the haemagglutinin protein expressed on the surface of the influenza virus. The epitopes recognized by antibodies (and B cell receptors) are accessible on the exposed parts

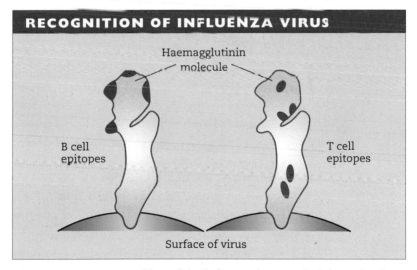

RECOGNITION OF INFLUENZA VIRUS

Haemagglutinin
molecule

B cell
epitopes

T cell
epitopes

Surface of virus

Fig. 2.7 Immune recognition of the influenza haemagglutinin molecule. The dark shading indicates the regions of the antigen recognized by B cells (and antibodies) or by T cells.

of the native molecule. By contrast, as a result of antigen processing, peptides which can associate with HLA molecules and be recognized by specific T cell receptors may originate from internal, as well as external, regions of the haemagglutinin protein.

The HLA system and its proteins

Although the physiological role of cell surface glycoproteins encoded within the **major histocompatibility complex** (MHC) is to present antigenic determinants to T cells, these molecules were initially identified by their role in transplant rejection. Indeed, they were found to play the most significant (*major*) role in determining whether a tissue transplant is recognized as foreign or not (*histocompatibility*).

Considerable interest in the biochemical uniqueness of the individual followed the introduction of organ transplantation in the 1960s. Although blood group antigen systems were already well defined it soon became clear that the individual tissue type was of paramount importance in determining the rate and severity of graft rejection. Tissue exchanged between genetically identical members of the same species is tolerated indefinitely whereas the exchange of tissue between genetically different members of the same species, and between members of different species, are both followed by the development of graft-reactive T cells and antibodies culminating in rejection of the foreign tissue. (The discrimination between self and foreign material is presented as a cardinal feature of the immune system on p. 7, and the details of tissue transplant rejection are considered in Chapter 18.) The MHC genes exist in a large number of alternative (allelic) forms in different individuals (i.e. they exhibit **polymorphism**). This results in significant differences in the amino acid sequences of MHC proteins from one individual to another. It is these differences that permit tissue transplants between individuals to be recognized as foreign by the recipient's lymphocytes.

THE STRUCTURE OF HLA MOLECULES

The unravelling of the human MHC has largely been achieved by documenting protein variations on the surfaces of peripheral blood leucocytes; hence the term **human leucocyte antigen** (HLA) system. Multiple pregnancies or blood transfusions often induce antibodies to these HLA proteins because of the allelic differences between mother and fetus or donor and recipient, and sera from such individuals have been used to type for these proteins. This is why HLA proteins are referred to as 'antigens'.

There are two main forms of HLA glycoproteins called **class I** and **class II**. HLA class I and class II molecules are made up of different types of polypeptide chains but they are both members of the immunoglobulin superfamily (Fig. 2.3). Their overall three-dimensional structures are similar and they both bind antigenic peptides for presentation to T cell receptors (Fig. 2.8). The roles of HLA class I and class II in different types of T cell responses are described in Chapter 3.

HLA class I glycoproteins are expressed on the surface of almost all nucleated cells. They consist of a large α polypeptide chain (molecular weight 45 000 daltons) and a smaller polypeptide of 12 000 daltons known as β_2-microglobulin (Fig. 2.8). The former contains three domains designated α_1, α_2 and α_3 with the lowermost part of the α chain extending through the cell membrane into the cytoplasm. The single domain of β_2-microglobulin associates non-covalently with the α chain. The α_3 domain and β_2-microglobulin are proximal to the cell membrane and are structurally related to immunoglobulin constant domains (Fig. 2.3). The α_1 and α_2 domains are distal to the cell membrane and together form an antigen binding groove, the walls of which are two α-helices lying across a platform of β-pleated sheet (Fig. 2.9a). The groove can accommodate an antigenic peptide of eight or nine amino acids (Fig. 2.9a) and a T cell receptor can bind simultaneously to the exposed surface of the epitope and the regions of the HLA molecule around the perimeter of the groove (Fig. 2.8).

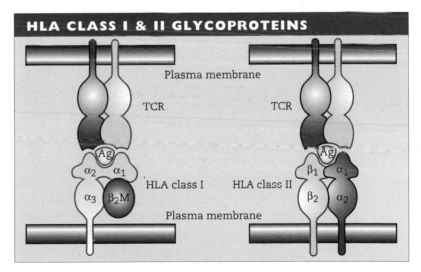

HLA CLASS I & II GLYCOPROTEINS

Plasma membrane

TCR   TCR

Ag   Ag

α_2 α_1 β_1 α_1

HLA class I   HLA class II

α_3 β_2M β_2 α_2

Plasma membrane

Fig. 2.8 The structure of HLA class I and II glycoproteins, and their interactions with antigenic determinants (Ag) and T cell receptors (TCR).

THE PEPTIDE BINDING GROOVES

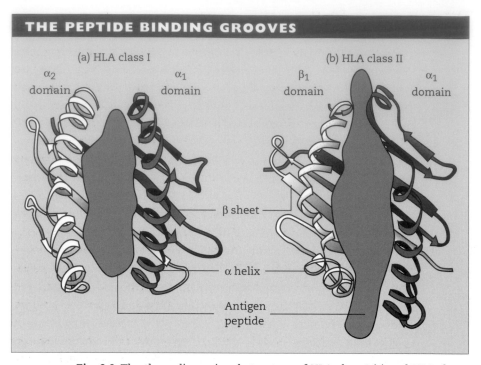

Fig. 2.9 The three-dimensional structure of HLA class I (a) and HLA class II (b) antigen peptide binding grooves which are formed by two α-helices lying on a platform of β-pleated sheet. The HLA class II binding groove has open ends and can accommodate longer antigenic peptides than the HLA class I binding groove with closed ends.

    The expression of HLA class II molecules is mainly confined to cells directly involved in immune responses, i.e. macrophages, other antigen-presenting cells (e.g. dendritic cells and Langerhans cells), B cells and activated T cells. HLA class II molecules are heterodimers of α and β polypeptide chains (33 000 and 28 000 daltons, respectively); each chain contains two polypeptide domains and traverses the cell membrane (Fig. 2.8). As with class I proteins, the two domains of HLA class II molecules proximal to the cell membrane (α_2 and β_2) show marked structural homology to other members of the immunoglobulin superfamily (Fig. 2.3). The distal domains (α_1 and β_1) form an antigen-binding groove similar to that of HLA class I molecules, except that the groove of HLA class II molecules has open ends so that longer antigenic peptides of 12 to 20 amino acids can be accommodated (Fig. 2.9b).

THE HLA COMPLEX OF GENES

The genes encoding HLA molecules form a cluster or complex of loci on chromosome 6 (Fig. 2.10). The first genetic loci encoding HLA molecules to be described were HLA-A and HLA-B followed by HLA-C. These genes encode the α chains of three class I molecules that are expressed on most cells (β_2-microglobulin is encoded elsewhere in the genome). Other class I genes have been identified to the right of HLA-A and include HLA-E, HLA-F and HLA-G. Their functions are unknown but all three are probably expressed to a limited extent, e.g. HLA-G can be detected on placental extravillous trophoblast during fetal gestation.

Three HLA class II molecules called HLA-DP, HLA-DQ and HLA-DR are encoded by genes for their α and β chains within the HLA complex (Fig. 2.10). The HLA-DR locus contains three functional genes: one α and two β genes, whereas the HLA-DQ and HLA-DP loci each have genes encoding one α and one β chain. The significance of other similar loci found within the class II region of the HLA complex is not yet clear.

The HLA complex also contains genes coding for other immunological components (Fig. 2.10). Within the HLA class II region are genes encoding proteasome components (LMP-1 and LMP-2) and peptide transporter proteins (Tap 1 and Tap 2) involved in one of the antigen processing pathways (see Chapter 4). Within what is termed the HLA class III region, there are also genes coding for complement proteins C2, factor B (Bf) and C4 (see Chapter 7), and the cytokines tumour necrosis factor and lymphotoxin (see Chapter 5).

HLA POLYMORPHISM

The genes for both HLA class I and class II molecules exist in a much larger number of allelic forms than is the case for most tissue components, and are therefore said to be **polymorphic**. The regions of the HLA molecules in which this variability mainly occurs form the antigen-binding groove which interacts with both antigenic determinants and the antigen receptors of T cells. It is for these reasons that the MHC molecules, expressed in tissue transplanted from one individual to another, are recognized as foreign by T cells of the recipient leading to an anti-graft immune response (see Chapter 18). By contrast, T cells which would react with self HLA in the absence of a foreign antigen are eliminated as part of the censoring process which occurs in the thymus (see p. 45).

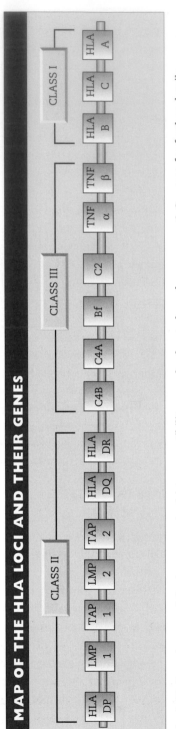

Fig. 2.10 Genetic map of the human major histocompatibility complex located on chromosome 6. See text for further details.

HLA & IMMUNE RESPONSIVENESS

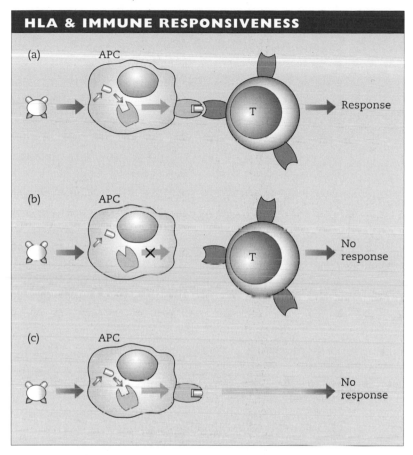

Fig. 2.11 Possible ways in which HLA molecules may influence immune responsiveness. Antigen is processed in an antigen presenting cell (APC) and antigen peptide interacts with the binding groove of an HLA molecule. This complex is transported to the cell surface where it can stimulate a T cell with receptors specific for the antigen (a). No response will occur if the HLA binding groove has a structure incompatible for association with the antigen peptide (b), or no T cells are available with receptors specific for this antigen–HLA combination (c).

Because allelic HLA molecules have differences in their binding grooves, they show preferences for interaction with particular antigenic peptides and T cell receptors. In extreme cases, an individual may be unable to make an immune response to a particular antigenic determinant because this peptide may not bind to the MHC molecules of the individual (Fig. 2.11b); alternatively, T cells capable of recognizing the MHC–antigen combination may have been deleted during T cell development in the thymus (see Chapter 3) because this particular combination looks very similar to tissue components of the individual, i.e. the T cells would be autoreactive (Fig. 2.11c). By contrast, other individuals expressing different MHC alleles may mount good responses to the determinant because it binds well to their MHC molecules and specific T cells are available to recognize it (Fig. 2.11a). This may help to explain why the major histocompatibility system has evolved extensive polymorphism: it ensures that at least some members of a population will be able to make a good immune response to any possible antigen, so it is unlikely that a pathogen could arise to which no individuals can mount an effective immune response. In view of these considerations, it is not surprising that many immunopathological diseases are associated with particular HLA types (see Chapter 16).

KEY POINTS

1 Antigens that induce immune responses are termed immunogens whereas those that induce non-responsiveness are known as tolerogens.

2 The specificity and affinity of interaction between an antigen receptor and an antigenic determinant (epitope) are dependent on complementarity of shape and charge.

3 The antigen receptors of B and T cells are related to other members of the immunoglobulin superfamily and the B cell receptor is a cell-bound form of secreted immunoglobulin.

4 The specificity of an immune response is ensured by the clonal selection of lymphocytes whose receptors bind the antigen with high affinity.

5 B cell antigen receptors and antibodies can bind antigen in its native, unmodified form, recognizing accessible surface epitopes. T cell receptors recognize antigenic peptides bound to HLA molecules expressed on the surface of antigen presenting cells or target cells: this requires processing (fragmentation) of the antigen, and epitopes may be derived from any part of the antigen.

6 HLA class I and HLA class II molecules are also members of the immunoglobulin superfamily and possess a groove which accommodates antigenic peptides for presentation to T cells.

7 There are three major class I molecules (HLA-A, -B, and -C) and three major class II molecules (HLA-DP, -DQ and -DR) encoded by genes within the HLA complex on chromosome 6.

8 HLA class I and class II genes exist in a large number of allelic forms (i.e. they are polymorphic). Each of them preferentially binds different antigenic peptides and this causes variation in immune responsiveness to particular antigens between different individuals.

Further reading

Bjorkman P.J., Saper M.A., Samraoui B., Bennett W.S., Strominger J.L. & Wiley D.C. (1987) Structure of the human class I histocompatibility antigen, HLA-A2. *Nature*, **329**, 506–512.

Bjorkman P.J., Saper M.A., Samraoui B., Bennett W.S., Strominger J.L. & Wiley D.C. (1987) The foreign antigen binding site and T cell recognition regions of class I histocompatibility antigens. *Nature*, **329**, 512–518.

Brown J.H., Jardetzky T.S., Gorga J.C., Stern L.J., Urban R.G., Strominger, J.L. & Wiley D.C. (1993) 3-Dimensional structure of the human class-II histocompatibility antigen HLA-DR1. *Nature*, **364**, 33–39.

Campbell R.D. & Trowsdale J. (1993) Map of the major histocompatibility complex. *Immunology Today*, **14**, 349–352.

Janeway C.A. (1994) How the immune system recognises invaders. In *Life, Death and the Immune System: Scientific American: A Special Issue*. W.H. Freeman, New York.

O'Brien C. (1995) Taking a first look at a T cell receptor. *Science*, **267**, 1906.

Rammensee H.-G., Falk K. & Rotzschke O. (1993) MHC molecules as peptide receptors. *Current Opinion in Immunology*, **5**, 35–44.

Stern L.J., Brown J.H., Jardetzky T.S., Gorga J.C., Urban R.G., Strominger J.L. & Wiley D.C. (1994) Crystal-structure of the human class-II MHC protein HLA-DR1 complexed with an influenza-virus peptide. *Nature*, **368**, 215–221.

CHAPTER 3

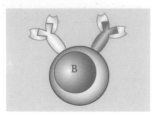

Lymphocyte Development and Differentiation

Little was known about the function of lymphocytes until the early 1960s when experiments performed by Gowans demonstrated that the lymphocyte was the immunocompetent cell without which the immune system lost its ability to recognize and respond to antigen. He showed that rats depleted of their lymphocytes by continuous thoracic duct drainage failed to reject foreign grafts and lost the ability to develop delayed hypersensitivity reactions and antibody responses. Each of these activities could be restored by returning the lymphocytes intravenously. Thus, lymphocytes are the cells responsible for conferring on the immune response the cardinal features of specificity, memory and self-discrimination.

The main features of lymphocyte development and differentiation are depicted in Fig. 3.1. Lymphocytes are derived from haemopoietic stem cells present, sequentially during ontogeny, in the yolk sac, liver and bone marrow. Lymphoid stem cells, like the precursors of the myeloid and erythroid lineages, are replenished from the **pluripotent stem cells** throughout life.

The primitive lymphoid cells which originate from bone marrow develop into two major lymphocyte populations. Some lymphocytes require a period of differentiation in the thymus and are called **T cells**. In birds, the other lymphocytes were found to differentiate in a lymphoid component of the hind gut—the Bursa of Fabricius—and were named **B cells**. Mammalian B cells, however, continue to differentiate in the bone marrow and emerge as mature lymphocytes. Bone marrow and thymus, being tissues in which lymphocytes constantly arise and develop throughout life, are known as **primary lymphoid organs**.

Mature lymphocytes leave the primary lymphoid organs and circulate

LYMPHOCYTE DIFFERENTIATION PATHWAYS

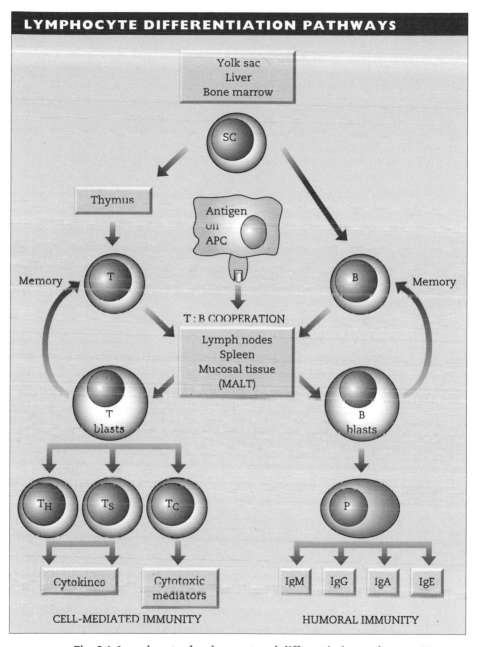

Fig. 3.1 Lymphocyte development and differentiation pathways. SC, stem cell; APC, antigen presenting cell; P, plasma cell; Ig, immunoglobulins: T_H, T_S and T_C, T lymphocytes with helper, suppressor and cytotoxic activities, respectively.

round the body and migrate through lymphocyte-rich tissues where lymphocyte activation is most likely to occur. These **secondary lymphoid organs** include lymph nodes, the white pulp of the spleen and mucosa-associated lymphoid tissue (MALT). B and T cells preferentially home to different parts of these tissues known, respectively, as B- and T-dependent areas.

B cell development

The earliest cells of the B lymphocyte lineage can be detected in fetal liver and are present in bone marrow throughout life (Fig. 3.1). The progenitor cells committed to this lineage randomly select variable region genes encoding the combining site of their antigen receptors and their secreted antibodies. The variety and arrangement of these genes is such that a vast number of different specificities (of the order of 10^8) can be generated within an individual (see p. 89), and the immune system can thus recognize many different antigens. However, all the antigen receptors of a single B cell have identical combining sites.

B cell antigen receptors and secreted antibodies occur as five **immunoglobulin classes**, designated IgM, IgD, IgG, IgA and IgE, which differ in the amino acid sequences of their heavy chains (see Chapter 6). The B cell precursors produce IgM heavy chains which can be detected in their cytoplasm. These are known as **pre-B cells** and they give rise to immature B cells which additionally produce light chains and express surface IgM.

B cell precursors require a variety of signals to guide them along the developmental pathway: these are provided by bone marrow stromal cells through surface and secreted molecules. However, some B cell precursors do not emerge from this pathway, but undergo a process of programmed cell death called **apoptosis** in which they degrade their own DNA. This may be because they do not rearrange the genes to encode functional antigen receptors (as described in Chapter 6). Alternatively, they may generate receptors which are specific for tissue components in their surroundings: binding these self-antigens triggers their deletion and thus helps to limit autoreactivity.

B cell activation and maturation

Most of the mature, unactivated (i.e. virgin) B cells which leave the bone marrow express both IgM and IgD on their surface: they are small cells, with only a thin rim of cytoplasm. The activation of B cells by most protein antigens requires help from T cells, which is facilitated by the expression of HLA class II molecules by B cells. Such responses are said to be **thymus-dependent** in view of their requirement for thymus-derived T cells. By contrast, some antigens (particularly certain carbohydrates and glycolipids) are able to stimulate B cells directly without the involvement of T cells, and are therefore called **thymus-independent**. A feature of such antigens is that they possess repeating antigenic determinants which enable them to cross-link the receptors of B cells to which they are specifically bound. Certain bacterial components (e.g. bacterial flagellin) have this property.

When activated by antigen, B cells enlarge and become **lymphoblasts** (Fig. 3.1). Some of their progeny mature into **plasma cells** which lack surface immunoglobulin, but synthesize large quantities of immuno-globulin molecules which are secreted as free antibody: the plasma cells have highly developed arrays of rough endoplasmic reticulum. Other B lymphoblasts revert to a resting state and form a **memory population** specific for the antigen which induced the primary response. It is these cells which, upon re-exposure to the same or a very similar cross-reactive antigen, generate a rapid and more vigorous secondary response, as exemplified in Fig. 1.1.

Virgin B cells express IgM and IgD but lose surface IgD expression following stimulation by antigen. Memory B cells also lack this class of immunoglobulin. Some of the B cells activated in a primary response mature into IgM-secreting plasma cells, but others, including many which become memory cells, switch the class of immunoglobulin they synthesize (to IgG, IgA or IgE) with little or no change in their antigenic specificity (Fig. 3.2). Thus, the majority of antibodies produced in a secondary response are of classes other than IgM. The immunoglobulin gene rearrangements which enable variable domains to be combined with different heavy chain constant regions in the various immunoglobulin classes are described in Chapter 6.

T cell development and education

The precursors of T lymphocytes leave the bone marrow at a very early stage of their development and migrate to the thymus (Fig. 3.1), which they enter at the outer margin of the cortex, and are then known as **thymocytes**. The thymic cortex is densely packed with actively proliferating, immature thymocytes, whereas the inner medulla is more sparsely populated by mature cells (derived from cortical thymocytes) which are destined to migrate to secondary lymphoid tissues. The

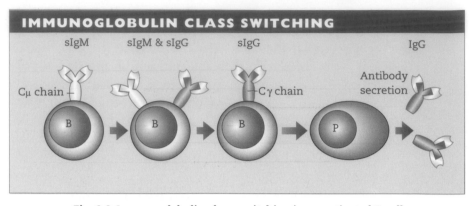

Fig. 3.2 Immunoglobulin class-switching in an activated B cell exemplified by a change from IgM to IgG production. This involves switching the C_H domains expressed, while the V_H domain and light chain (V_L and C_L domains) are unchanged. P, plasma cell.

medulla also contains complex aggregates of epithelial cells — Hassall's corpuscles — the function of which is unknown.

Soon after entering the thymus, each thymocyte starts to express the α and β polypeptide chains of its T cell receptors (TCR) specific for antigen plus HLA (p. 29), having randomly selected variable region genes from the large number available in a manner analogous to that employed by B cells in generating their surface immunoglobulins (see p. 89). Thus, although all the antigen combining sites of a single thymocyte are identical, these cells collectively express a large repertoire of specificities. Associated with the TCR on the cell surface is a molecule called **CD3** which transmits signals into the cell when the TCR binds to antigen plus HLA. (Details of the CD nomenclature of cell surface molecules are given in Table 3.1.)

At this stage, each thymocyte also bears two surface glycoproteins called **CD4** and **CD8**, which are members of the immunoglobulin superfamily (see Fig. 2.3). However, cells which survive to become mature T cells continue to express only one of these two molecules: normally, about 65% of T cells in the blood circulation are CD4$^+$ and 35% are CD8$^+$, although this bias is reversed in some diseases. T cells expressing CD4 always recognize antigen in association with HLA class II molecules, whereas CD8$^+$ T cells interact with antigen in association with HLA class I. This is because, as illustrated in Fig. 3.3, CD4 molecules interact with the β_2-domain of HLA class II, and CD8 with the α_3-domain of HLA class I (i.e. at sites distinct from the antigen binding groove engaged by the TCR) thus enhancing the overall interaction between the T cell and the antigen bearing cell.

CD MOLECULES

CD designation	Function/Description
CD2	Receptor for LFA-3 (CD58)
CD3	TCR-associated triggering molecule
CD4	HLA class II binding molecule
CD8	HLA class I binding molecule
CD11/CD18	The two chains of leucocyte integrins: receptors for ICAM-1 (CD54)
CD25	Receptor for interleukin-2
CD28	Costimulatory molecule on T cells: receptor for B7/BB1 (CD80)
CD40	Costimulatory molecule on B cells: receptor for CD40-ligand
CD49/CD29	The two chains of the VLA integrins: receptors for VCAM-1 (CD106) and connective tissue proteins
CD62	Selectins

The CD nomenclature has been devised to catalogue cell surface molecules as they are identified and characterized. These molecules are often initially defined on certain cell types by producing monoclonal antibodies (see p. 99) which bind to them specifically. CD stands for 'cluster of differentiation', referring to the *cluster* of monoclonal antibodies which define a particular *differentiation* molecule. Over 130 CD molecules have been designated. Some examples referred to in this chapter and in Chapter 4 are listed here.

Table 3.1 Examples of CD molecules.

INTERACTION OF CD8 & CD4 WITH HLA

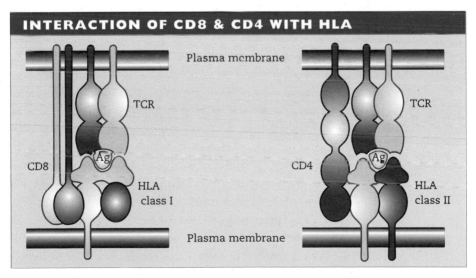

Fig. 3.3 A schematic representation of the interaction between a CD8+ T cell and antigenic determinant (Ag) bound to HLA class I, and a CD4+ T cell and antigenic determinant bound to HLA class II. TCR, T cell receptor.

T cells are central to the activation and regulation of immune responses. It is therefore important that they interact efficiently with foreign antigens presented on self-HLA molecules, but do not react against other components of 'self'. These restrictions on the T cell repertoire of antigenic specificities are determined by the selective development of precursors in the thymus — a process known as **T cell education** — during which more than 95% of developing thymocytes are eliminated.

The stromal framework of the thymus includes an epithelial component, which develops from the third and fourth pharyngeal pouches, and bone marrow-derived interdigitating dendritic cells and macrophages. The stromal cells express both HLA class I and class II molecules whose antigen binding grooves bear 'self' peptides (derived by natural degradation of the body's own proteins). The interaction of a thymocyte's TCR with these cells plays a large part in determining whether or not it will be selected to become a fully developed T cell (Fig. 3.4).

Any thymocytes which do not interact with the stromal cells, either because they have failed to develop functional TCR or because their TCR cannot bind to self-HLA, undergo programmed cell death by apoptosis. Thymocytes whose TCR bind with high avidity to HLA molecules on stromal cells (thereby showing specificity for the self-antigens) are also eliminated by apoptosis.

The thymocytes which are selected for continued development are those whose TCR show low avidity for stromal HLA molecules bearing self-peptides, inferring that they would bind more strongly to foreign peptides bound to self-HLA. Furthermore, those thymocytes whose TCRs interact with HLA class I maintain expression of CD8 but lose CD4, and *vice versa* for those interacting with HLA class II. Thus, the medullary thymocytes, which have survived passage through the cortex and which become mature recirculating T cells, express either CD4 or CD8 and are mainly specific for foreign antigens bound to self-HLA molecules.

T cell subpopulations

Mature T cells show heterogeneity in their functional properties as well as in their expression of CD4 and CD8. Some T cells cooperate with B cells, helping them to respond to antigen, resulting in B cell differentiation into antibody-secreting plasma cells. These are termed **helper T cells** (T_H) (Fig. 3.1). The help provided by T_H to B cells is dependent both on direct interactions and on the T cells secreting activating molecules called

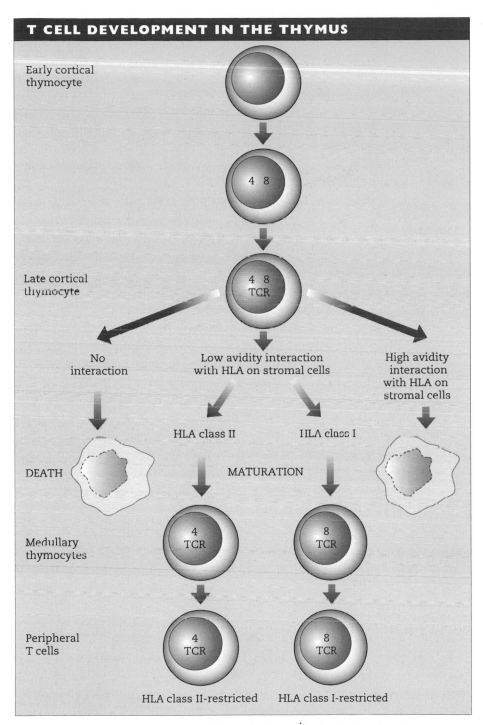

Fig. 3.4 Stages of T cell differentiation and selection in the thymus.

cytokines which bind to, and stimulate, B cells (see Chapter 5). Cytokines also attract and activate other lymphocytes and monocytes, as seen in the delayed hypersensitivity type of inflammatory reaction (discussed in Chapter 15). There is evidence that distinct subpopulations of T cells preferentially promote cell-mediated immunity (T_H1) or stimulate antibody production (T_H2) based on the types of cytokines they produce (see Table 3.2 and Chapter 5).

Other T cells are able to kill virus-infected or allogeneic cells, i.e. cells expressing foreign determinants on their surface, and are called **cytotoxic T cells** (T_C) (Fig. 3.1). Most T_H express CD4, whereas T_C are mainly $CD8^+$. This correlation of function with phenotype is not absolute, however, for a minority of $CD4^+$ T cells have cytotoxic activity.

Some T cells are able to suppress immune responses and have therefore been designated **suppressor T cells** (T_S). However, rather than T_S being a distinct subpopulation, it appears more likely that suppression is an aspect of other T cell activities. For example, T_H1 and T_H2 cells exert mutual inhibition through the cytokines they produce (see Table 3.2 and Chapter 5). Another mechanism involves T cells which have become unresponsive (termed **anergy** – see p. 55) causing suppression by competing with responsive T cells for binding to antigen presenting cells and for cytokines.

LARGE GRANULAR LYMPHOCYTES

Up to 15 per cent of blood lymphocytes express neither TCR nor surface immunoglobulin and most of these cells are larger than resting T or B cells, having more cytoplasm which also contains azurophilic granules. They are known as large granular lymphocytes and are cytotoxic to

PROPERTIES OF T_H1 AND T_H2 CELLS		
Property	**T_H1**	**T_H2**
Cytokines produced	Interleukin-2 Interferon-γ	Interleukin-4 Interleukin-10
Cell types helped	Macrophages Cytotoxic T cells	B cells
Immunity generated	Cell-mediated	Antibody-mediated
Cells suppressed	T_H2 cells	T_H1 cells

Table 3.2 The properties of T_H1 and T_H2 cells.

certain tumour cells and virally infected cells, mediating **natural killer** activity and **antibody-dependent cellular cytotoxicity** (see Chapter 10).

KEY POINTS

1 Stem cells in the bone marrow give rise to precursors which, in the case of B cells, mature in the bone marrow. T cell precursors migrate to the thymus for their development. The sites in which lymphocytes develop are known as primary lymphoid organs.

2 Antigen receptor diversity is generated during lymphocyte development by random selection of variable region genes in different lymphocytes.

3 Lymphocyte precursors which recognize self-antigens are deleted through interactions with stromal cells, whereas those which can recognize foreign antigens develop fully. T cells are also selected for expression of CD8 or CD4, which restricts them to recognize antigen associated with HLA class I or class II, respectively.

4 Mature lymphocytes migrate to secondary lymphoid tissues (lymph node, spleen, mucosa-associated lymphoid tissues) which are the main sites of stimulation by antigens.

5 When activated by antigen, a lymphocyte becomes a proliferating lymphoblast, some of whose progeny become memory cells, and others effector cells. B lymphoblasts can switch the class of immunoglobulin which they express.

6 Antibody-secreting plasma cells arise from B cells, while effector T cells have regulatory (T_H, T_S) or cytotoxic (T_C) functions.

Further reading

Davis M.M. & Bjorkman P.J. (1988) T-cell antigen receptor genes and T-cell recognition. *Nature*, **334**, 395–402.

Hogquist K.A., Jameson S.C. & Bevan M.J. (1994) The ligand for positive selection of T lymphocytes in the thymus. *Current Opinion in Immunology*, **6**, 273–278.

Law C.-L. & Clark E.A. (1994) Cell–cell interactions that regulate the development of B-lineage cells. *Current Opinion in Immunology*, **6**, 238–247.

Marrack P. & Kappler J.W. (1994) How the immune system recognizes the body. In *Life, Death and the Immune System: Scientific American: A Special Issue*. W.H. Freeman, New York.

Murphy D.B. (1993) T cell mediated immunosuppression. *Current Opinion in Immunology*, **5**, 411–417.

Owen M.J. & Jenkinson E. (1993) Ontogeny of the immune system. In Lachmann P.J., Peters D.K., Rosen F.S. & Walport M.J. eds, *Clinical Aspects of Immunology*, 5th edn. Blackwell Scientific Publications, Oxford.

Parker D.C. (1993) B lymphocytes and B lymphocyte activation. In Lachmann P.J., Peters D.K., Rosen F.S. & Walport M.J. eds, *Clinical Aspects of Immunology*, 5th edn. Blackwell Scientific Publications, Oxford.

Scott P. (1993) Selective differentiation of CD4$^+$ T helper cell subsets. *Current Opinion in Immunology*, **5**, 391–397.

Terhorst C. & Regueiro J.R. (1993) T cell activation. In Lachmann P.J., Peters D.K., Rosen F.S. & Walport M.J. eds, *Clinical Aspects of Immunology*, 5th edn. Blackwell Scientific Publications, Oxford.

Weissman I.L. & Cooper M.D. (1994) How the immune system develops. In *Life, Death and the Immune System: Scientific American: A Special Issue*. W.H. Freeman, New York.

CHAPTER 4

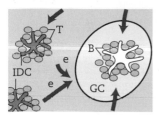

Lymphocyte Interactions and the Lymphoid System

Both the activation and functions of lymphocytes require them to interact with each other and with other cell types, while specific recognition of antigens triggers and focuses these activities. The opportunities for these interactions are maximized by the recirculation of lymphocytes throughout the body and by their homing to secondary lymphoid tissues.

Cytotoxic T cells

An important function of T_C cells is to eliminate other cells which could be detrimental to the body as a whole, e.g. virus-infected cells. Since most cell types can become infected by different types of viruses, it is important that all cells are subject to surveillance by T_C. This is achieved by the expression of CD8 by most T_C which restricts them to the recognition of antigen associated with HLA class I, and the fact that most cell types of the body do express HLA class I molecules (see Table 4.1). Figure 4.1

T CELL TYPES & HLA MOLECULES

T cell type	HLA restriction	HLA distribution	Immune function
CD8+ T_C	Class I	Most cells	Surveillance of all cells, e.g. for viral infection
CD4+ T_H	Class II	Mainly immune cells	Controlled and appropriate way activation of immune cells

Table 4.1 Relationship between T cell phenotype, HLA restriction and function.

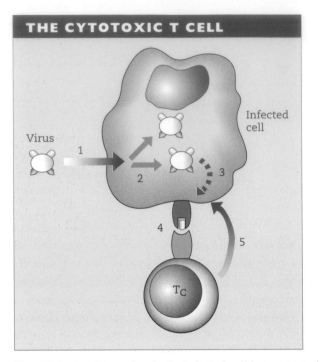

THE CYTOTOXIC T CELL

Fig. 4.1 Recognition of a virally infected cell by a cytotoxic T cell (T_C). The stages represented are: (1) entry of the virus into the target cell; (2) replication of the virus; (3) processing of viral proteins to generate antigenic determinants which associate with HLA class I molecules; (4) presentation of the antigen–HLA complex for recognition by a specific CD8+ T_C; (5) killing of the infected cell by the T_C.

illustrates this recognition of a virus infected **target cell** by a T_C. Viruses do not possess the biological machinery necessary to replicate their own genetic material, and can only proliferate by infecting cells and subverting cellular components for their own ends. T_C prevent this replication by specifically recognizing and killing virus infected cells: this would not be achieved if T_C had receptors which could directly recognize free viral particles as antigens.

The route or **processing pathway** whereby antigenic peptides are generated for binding to HLA class I molecules is shown in Fig. 4.2. These peptides are produced endogenously, being generated from proteins synthesized in the cytosol (i.e. the cytoplasmic fluid) of the cell, and signal to the T_C that the target cell is a source of antigens (e.g. infectious viral particles) and should therefore be killed. Protein antigens present in the cytoplasm are degraded in an enzyme complex called a **proteasome** and

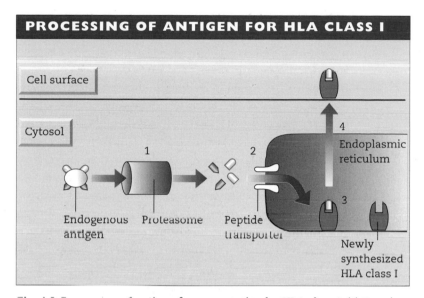

PROCESSING OF ANTIGEN FOR HLA CLASS I

Cell surface

Cytosol

4
Endoplasmic
reticulum

1

2

3

Endogenous   Proteasome   Peptide
antigen   transporter

Newly
synthesized
HLA class I

Fig. 4.2 Processing of antigen for presentation by HLA class I. (1) Protein antigens present in the cytoplasm are degraded in an enzyme complex called a proteasome; (2) some of the peptides generated are transferred to the endoplasmic reticulum via peptide transporter proteins; (3) peptides of appropriate length (8 or 9 amino acids) and amino acid sequence associate with newly synthesized HLA class I molecules; (4) the peptide–HLA complexes are transported to the cell surface where they are available for recognition by T cells.

some of the peptides generated are transferred to the endoplasmic reticulum via **peptide transporter proteins**. Peptides of appropriate length (8 or 9 amino acids) and amino acid sequence associate with newly synthesized HLA class I molecules. The HLA class I molecules serve as couriers to deliver fragments of the endogenous antigens to the cell surface and present them to specific T_C, thus focusing cytotoxic activity where it is most needed.

HELPER T CELLS

The role of T_H is to help other cells of the immune system, such as macrophages and B lymphocytes, to become activated in order to fulfil their effector functions. These cells express HLA class II molecules whereas most tissue cell types do not. T_H cells express CD4, thereby restricting them to the recognition of antigen associated with HLA class II and directing them to interact with these other cells of the immune system (see Table 4.1).

The processing pathway for antigens which associate with HLA class II molecules is shown in Fig. 4.3. This requires antigen to enter a cytoplasmic vesicle called an **endosome**, which occurs when exogenous antigen is engulfed by a process termed **endocytosis**. Peptides generated by enzymatic degradation of the antigen then associate with newly synthesized HLA class II molecules which migrate to the vacuole from the endoplasmic reticulum. The class II molecules then transport the peptides to the cell surface for presentation to T_H cells. T cells help macrophages when dealing with infectious microbes like mycobacteria or leishmania which the macrophages engulf. Mycobacterial peptides associated with HLA class II molecules can be presented at the macrophage surface for direct interaction with specific **T_H1 cells** (see Table 3.2). These can then activate the macrophages to kill mycobacteria (Fig. 4.4).

Macrophages and other antigen presenting cells (APC) stimulate the activity of the T_H cells with which they interact. In particular,

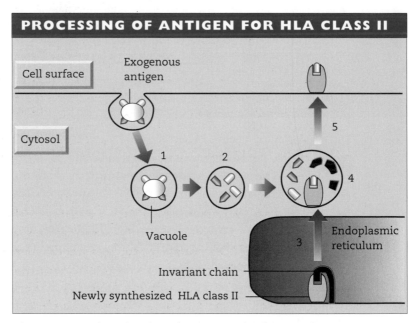

PROCESSING OF ANTIGEN FOR HLA CLASS II

Fig. 4.3 Processing of antigen for presentation by HLA class II.
(1) Endocytosis of exogenous protein antigen leads to its internalization into a vacuole; (2) enzymes entering the vacuole degrade the antigen;
(3) newly synthesized HLA class II molecules in the endoplasmic reticulum associate with the invariant chain and are transported to the vacuole; (4) the invariant chain is degraded and antigen peptides of the appropriate length and amino acid sequence associate with the class II molecules; (5) the peptide–HLA complexes are transported to the cell surface where they are available for recognition by T cells.

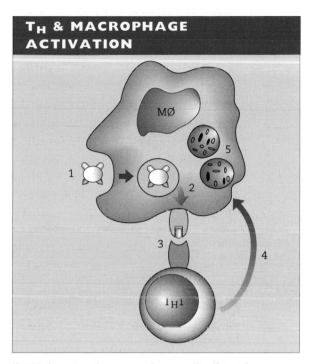

Fig. 4.4 Helper T cell (T$_H$) function for macrophage activation. The stages represented are: (1) phagocytosis of microbes into cytoplasmic vesicles; (2) processing and presentation of microbial antigens in association with HLA class II molecules; (3) interaction with a T$_H$1 cell; (4) activation of macrophages by cytokines secreted by the T$_H$1 cell (e.g. interferon-γ); (5) enhanced digestive activity of the macrophage results in destruction of the microbes.

interdigitating dendritic cells (IDC) are exceptionally good at presenting antigen to T$_H$ cells. Their name derives from the fact that they possess long finger-like cytoplasmic processes (dendrites) which enable them to interact with a large number of lymphocytes. Figure 4.5 illustrates the activation of a **T$_H$2 cell** (see Table 3.2) by an APC and the consequent ability of the T$_H$2 cell to stimulate antibody production by a B cell. This is facilitated by the B cell itself acting as an APC, presenting HLA class II-associated antigen to focus interaction with specific T$_H$2 cells. A feature of B cells which distinguishes them from other APCs is that they have surface receptors specific for antigen, i.e. surface immunoglobulin. Since these receptors bind specific antigen with high affinity, B cells are able to take up and present this antigen much more efficiently than other antigens which are not recognized by the surface receptors. However, in order for a B cell to be stimulated by a T cell, the epitope which will be recognized by the T cell must be physically linked to that bound by the surface receptors of the B cell. Only in this way will the T cell epitope be taken up efficiently by the B cell for processing and presentation to the T cell (Fig. 4.5).

COSTIMULATION OF LYMPHOCYTE ACTIVATION

Although the activation of lymphocytes is governed primarily by interactions with antigen and HLA, other stimuli are also required for efficient activation. Some are soluble mediators called **cytokines** (discussed in Chapter 5), while others involve adhesive interactions between surface

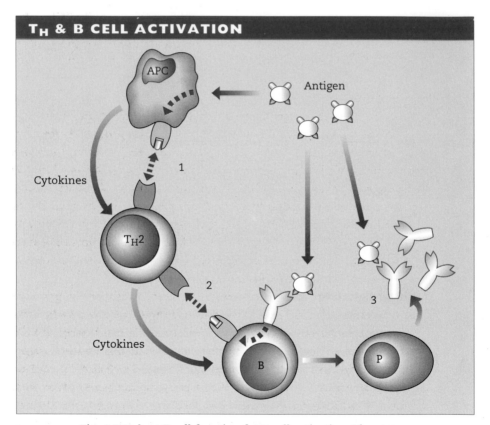

T_H & B CELL ACTIVATION

Fig. 4.5 Helper T cell function for B cell activation. The stages represented are: (1) antigen processing and presentation in association with HLA class II for recognition by a specific CD4+ T_H2 cell; (2) binding and processing of antigen by a specific B cell with HLA class II association for interaction with the T_H2 cell; (3) activation of the B cell results in the production of antibodies specific for the antigen. Cytokines also contribute to the activation processes (see Chapter 5). APC, antigen presenting cell; P, plasma cell.

ADHESION MOLECULES

	Receptor on lymphocyte	Ligand on interacting cell
T cells	CD4	HLA class II
	CD8	HLA class I
	CD28	CD80
	CD2	LFA-3
	VLA-4	VCAM-1
B cells	LFA-1	ICAM-1, -2 or -3
	CD40	CD40-Ligand

LFA, lymphocyte function-associated antigen; VLA, very late antigen; ICAM, intercellular adhesion molecule; VCAM, vascular cell adhesion molecule.

Table 4.2 Adhesion molecules involved in lymphocyte interaction.

molecules of the communicating cells (Table 4.2). In particular, the activation of T cells requires the binding of CD28 expressed on the T cell surface with CD80 which is expressed by APC such as activated macrophages, IDC and activated B cells. Antigen recognition by T cells in the absence of the CD28–CD80 interaction causes the T cells to become **anergic** (i.e. unresponsive) to further stimulation, or even to die by apoptosis. In a similar fashion, the antigen-specific activation of B cells by T cells requires the interaction of CD40 on the B cell surface with its ligand, CD40L (expressed by activated T cells) and without this interaction the B cell may undergo apoptosis.

Various other adhesion molecules can be involved in the interactions of T and B cells with each other and with other cell types, to facilitate lymphocyte activation (Table 4.2). These include the binding of CD2 (expressed by T cells) to LFA-3 (lymphocyte function-associated antigen-3), and LFA-1 to ICAM-1 (intercellular adhesion molecule-1). Furthermore, activated T cells express VLA-4 (very late antigen-4) which binds to VCAM-1 (vascular cell adhesion molecule-1). Adhesion molecules also play a role in leucocyte interactions with endothelial cells, as described on p. 156.

The lymphoid system

In order for lymphocytes to maintain constant surveillance for foreign antigens throughout the body, and to mount an efficient response when an antigen is detected, a dynamic and highly organized lymphoid system is required.

SECONDARY LYMPHOID TISSUES

Lymphoid tissues, e.g. lymph nodes, the white pulp of the spleen and mucosa-associated lymphoid tissue (MALT), are the main sites of lymphocyte activation by antigens. Both T and B lymphocytes actively recirculate and preferentially home to different parts of these tissues known, respectively, as T- and B-dependent areas.

Lymph nodes (see Fig. 4.6)

B lymphocytes are found predominantly in the outer cortex of lymph nodes which contains a number of dense aggregations of lymphocytes termed **follicles**. These enlarge during an active immune response to form **germinal centres** which contain large numbers of proliferating B lymphoblasts surrounded by a mantle of resting small B lymphocytes. T lymphocytes are diffusely present throughout the **paracortex** of the lymph node. The cooperative events which take place within lymph nodes to generate the antigen-specific activation of lymphocytes are outlined in Figs 4.6 and 4.8 and described on p. 60.

Fig. 4.6 Lymph node structure and lymphocyte activation. The lower diagram shows the overall structure of a lymph node with cortical aggregations of B lymphocytes into **follicles** (F) and **germinal centres** (GC) and subdivision of the medulla into **medullary cords** (MC) and **medullary sinuses** (MS). T lymphocytes are the predominant cell in the paracortex.

The upper diagram is an amplified inset of part of the cortex indicating the pathways by which antigen and lymphocytes gain access to the lymph node. This is either via **afferent lymphatics** (AL) and the **subcapsular sinus** (SCS) (a and c) or via the **post-capillary venules** (PCV) (b and d). Antigen in the form of immune complexes preferentially localizes to **follicular dendritic cells** (FDC) in the B cell-containing follicles or GC, whereas antigen transported by dendritic cells in lymph (and possibly blood) is presented to T helper cells in the paracortex which come into close contact with these **interdigitating dendritic cells** (IDC).

The process of T–B cooperation involves the approximation of these two kinds of cell in the paracortex culminating in the production of B lymphoblasts which migrate to the follicles (e) where they undergo further maturation and selection through interaction with antigen on follicular dendritic cells in the germinal centres before migrating (f) into the medullary cords where they can be detected as antibody-secreting cells.

Spleen

The T- and B-dependent areas of the spleen are confined to the white pulp: the follicles and marginal zones are mostly occupied by B cells whereas the periarteriolar sheath consists almost entirely of T cells.

MALT

Unencapsulated mucosa-associated lymphoid tissue or MALT (which includes **tonsils**, **Peyer's patches**, **appendix**, **bronchial** and **mam-**

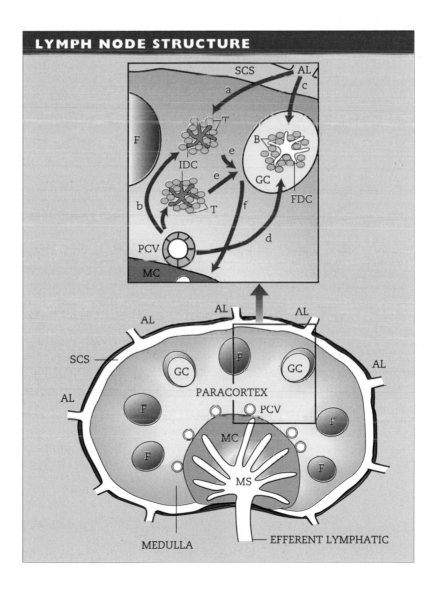

LYMPH NODE STRUCTURE

mary tissue), contains many follicles, but lymphocytes are also diffusely distributed in the subepithelial **lamina propria** of the intestine where only occasional follicles are present. Many of the lymphocytes in the lamina propria have the characteristics of large granular lymphocytes and the gut is also well endowed with its own variant of the mast cell, i.e. the mucosal mast cell. Many intestinal intraepithelial lymphocytes possess the $\gamma\delta$ type of antigen receptor (see p. 24).

Lymphocyte recirculation and homing

Once they have left the primary lymphoid organs, mature lymphocytes continually recirculate between the blood, body tissues and secondary lymphoid organs (Fig. 4.7). There is a modest, but steady, transit of lymphocytes across the venules of most tissues in the resting state. These cells migrate into **afferent lymphatics** and gain access to lymph nodes via the **marginal sinus** (Fig. 4.6). However, the majority of lymphocytes which enter lymph nodes do so directly from the blood supply of the nodes, within a specialized region of the postcapillary venules lined by activated **high endothelial cells**, these being enlarged, cuboidal cells, unlike the more common flat endothelium. Lymphocytes adhere to the high endothelial cells and migrate between them to enter the node. These processes are dependent on interactions between cell surface adhesion molecules, called **selectins** and **integrins**, and their coligands (discussed in more detail in Chapter 11).

Different lymphocytes preferentially home to different lymphoid organs, this being determined by the particular combinations of adhesion molecules expressed by lymphocytes and high endothelial cells. For example, lymphocytes which have been stimulated by antigen in one kind of lymphoid tissue (e.g. mucosal or non-mucosal) preferentially home back to the same kind of tissue. This is of value in defence against infections acquired by a particular route. It is relevant to the newborn in that mothers challenged intestinally with antigen develop antibody-secreting cells which migrate to mammary tissue and produce secretory IgA of relevant specificity in their milk.

Lymphocytes exit from lymph nodes via the **medulla** and **efferent lymphatics** to enter the blood circulation via the **thoracic duct** (Figs 4.6 & 4.7). The spleen has no lymphatic supply and splenic lymphocytes gain direct access to the circulation via the splenic vein.

The recirculation of lymphocytes (about 1–2 per cent per hour) enables the immune system continually to monitor the whole body for

LYMPHOCYTE RECIRCULATION

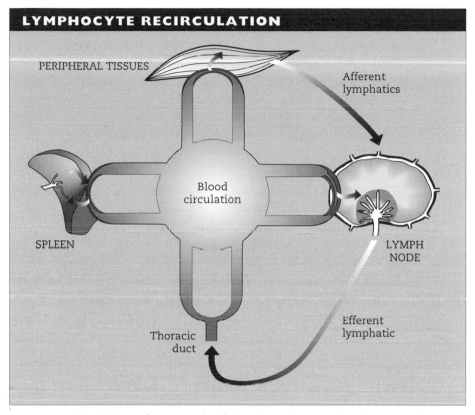

Fig. 4.7 Lymphocyte recirculation. Lymphocytes enter lymph nodes from the blood by crossing specialized 'high endothelium' in the postcapillary venules.

many different antigens, despite the relatively small number of lymphocytes specific for each. The homing to organized lymphoid tissues brings together the various lymphocytes and antigen presenting cells which must cooperate in order to mount an efficient immune response, as described in the next section.

Lymphocyte selection and maturation

The secondary lymphoid organs are the main sites of lymphocyte activation by antigen. The route of antigen access to the body determines the primary sites of interaction: antigenic material coming into contact with mucosal surfaces will localize to MALT, while blood-borne material is taken up by the spleen. Antigen in tissue fluids enters draining lymph nodes either as free antigen in the lymph, or bound to specialized cells. In the skin, for example, **Langerhans cells** bind antigen and transport it to lymph nodes where they become IDC which present antigen to T cells of the paracortex. When a lymph node is stimulated by antigen there is a general increase in lymphocyte uptake across the high endothelium. This influx is not selective for lymphocytes which recognize the antigen but those which interact with antigen are retained in the node where they become activated and proliferate. Several days later some of these cells enter the medulla and efferent lymph as blast cells and, later still, there is an efflux of memory cells into the circulation.

The processes of lymphocyte cooperation and maturation induced by antigen recognition in lymph nodes are illustrated in Figs 4.6 and 4.8. In the paracortex, T_H cells, activated by antigens presented on IDC, interact with specific B cells presenting the same antigens. The activated B cells then migrate to the adjacent follicles where they undergo rapid proliferation (as **centroblasts**) to form **germinal centres**. B cells with varying affinities for the antigen are generated by **somatic mutation** of their immunoglobulin variable domains (see Chapter 6). The **centrocytes** (as they are known at this stage) with highest affinity are selected for further maturation by interacting with antigen held for long periods on the surface of **follicular dendritic cells** (FDC) in the form of **immune complexes** with antibodies. The centrocytes with lower affinity for antigen, which do not interact with FDC, undergo apoptosis and die. (FDC, like IDC, have dendritic processes and are non-phagocytic but, in other respects, are very different. In accordance with their antigen presenting function for B cells but not T cells, FDC lack expression of HLA class II molecules.)

The selected B cells after immunoglobulin class switching, further proliferate leading to the formation of plasma cells and memory cells. These processes explain how the antigen specificity of a response is determined by **clonal selection** (see p. 26).

REGULATION OF LYMPHOCYTE RESPONSES

The ability of the adaptive immune system to switch off responses when they are no longer needed is essential for purposes of economy, to allow for responses to other antigens which may be encountered, and to prevent the benefits of eliminating an invading antigen being over-shadowed by unacceptable damage to self tissues (see Chapters 14–16). All immune responses can be regarded as a balance between help and suppression, but it is not clear why most start with help predominating and end with suppression to the fore. Clearance of the stimulating

B CELL MATURATION IN THE GERMINAL CENTRE

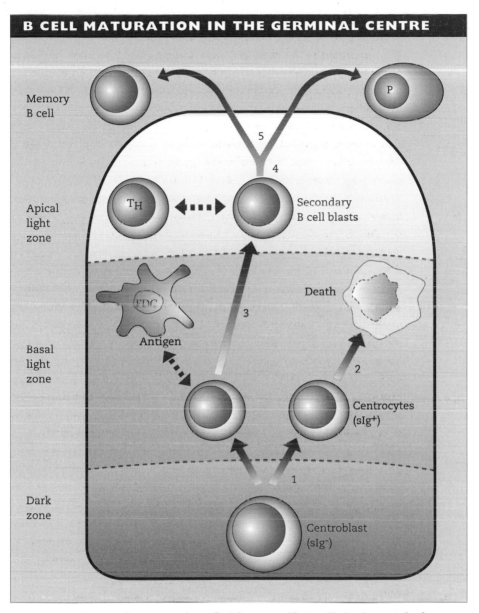

Fig. 4.8 The maturation of antigen-specific B cells in the germinal centre of a lymph node. (1) Clonal expansion and somatic mutation; (2) failure to interact with antigen on follicular dendritic cells (FDC) leads to cell death; (3) selection for further maturation is driven by interaction with antigen on FDC; (4) proliferation and isotype switching; (5) B memory cell development or maturation to plasma cells.

antigen should obviously contribute to the waning of a response, and some forms of antigen–antibody complexes inhibit lymphocyte activation. Much attention has focused on T cells which suppress immune responses by an inhibitory effect on the activity of T_H cells. However, as mentioned in Chapter 3, it is likely that T cell-mediated suppression can be achieved by a variety of mechanisms.

Laboratory methods

IDENTIFICATION AND ISOLATION OF LYMPHOCYTES

A variety of molecules expressed on the surface of lymphocytes are not found on other cell types. These **differentiation markers** are often utilized in the identification and isolation of lymphocytes. The CD nomenclature for these markers is outlined on p. 43. A number of techniques use antibodies (monoclonal or polyclonal, see p. 99) which specifically bind to a particular marker. For example, anti-CD3 antibodies specifically bind to T cells, but not to other leucocytes. If a fluorescent molecule (e.g. fluorescein or rhodamine) has been conjugated to the antibodies, the T cells can then be identified by the fluorescence observed in a UV microscope or detected in a **fluorescence activated cell sorter**, which will separate the fluorescent from the unlabelled cells (Fig. 4.9). The isolation of a particular type of lymphocyte can also be achieved by interaction with antibodies (against a surface marker) bound to a plastic dish (a technique called **panning**) or to particles (e.g. magnetic beads or red blood cells – known as **rosetting**) (Fig. 4.9). The CD2 molecules on T cells will bind to LFA-3 molecules on sheep red blood cells and this property is used in the formation of rosettes (Fig. 4.9).

The above techniques can be used to select cells positively, i.e. those that bind to a particular antibody, or to select negatively all the cells which are not bound. Another method for negative selection is to add complement (see Chapter 7), so that all the cells which have bound the antibody are lysed.

STIMULATION OF LYMPHOCYTES

Within a population of lymphocytes only a very small proportion specifically react to one particular antigen. These can be detected by the changes they undergo and the effects they mediate when stimulated by antigen. The activation of T lymphocytes results in metabolic activity and rapid proliferation, which can be quantified *in vitro* by the incorporation

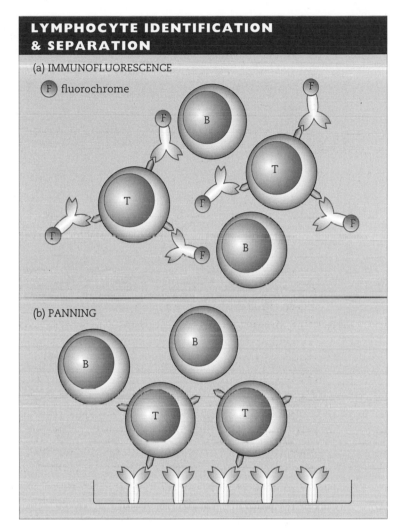

Fig. 4.9 Techniques for the identification and separation of lymphocytes, as applied to T cells. (a)–(c) show methods employing anti-T cell antibody (e.g. anti-CD3) with the antibody conjugated to a fluorescent probe (a), a plastic dish (b) or microscopic particles (c). The direct rosetting of T cells with sheep red blood cells (SRBC) is illustrated in (d) (Continued on p. 64)

of a radioactively labelled precursor into the newly synthesized DNA, RNA or protein. This is known as the **lymphocyte transformation test**.

The cytotoxic activity of T_C and large granular lymphocytes can be determined in the **chromium release assay**. Target cells are incubated

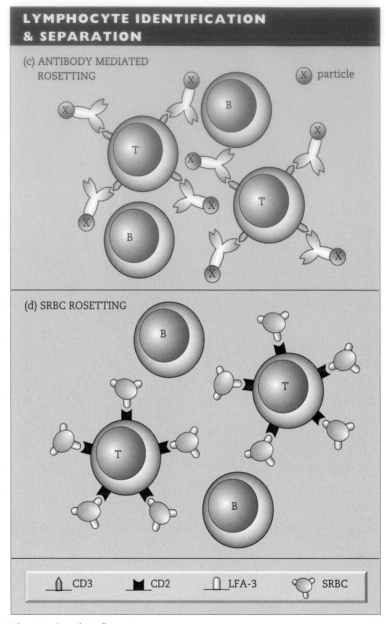

Fig. 4.9 (continued)

with a radioactive chromium compound which they take up into their cytoplasm. Lysis of the targets by killer cells can be measured by the release of radioactivity into the extracellular fluid.

The activation of B cells by antigen results in their maturation into

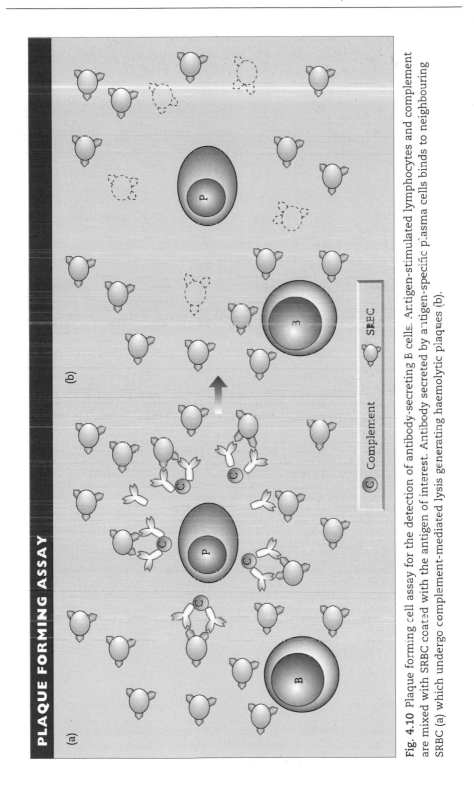

Fig. 4.10 Plaque forming cell assay for the detection of antibody-secreting B cells. Antigen-stimulated lymphocytes and complement are mixed with SRBC coated with the antigen of interest. Antibody secreted by antigen-specific plasma cells binds to neighbouring SRBC (a) which undergo complement-mediated lysis generating haemolytic plaques (b).

plasma cells, which can be detected by the specific antibodies they secrete. One means of doing this is by the **plaque forming cell assay**, illustrated in Fig. 4.10.

KEY POINTS

1 Cytotoxic function is associated with CD8⁺ T cells and HLA class I-associated antigen recognition. This facilitates T cell recognition and killing of tissue cells bearing antigens derived from cytosolic processing (e.g. following viral infection).

2 Helper function is associated with CD4⁺ T cells and HLA class II-associated antigen recognition. This facilitates T cell help by interaction with cells such as macrophages and B cells. The antigens are processed by endocytosis and degradation in cytoplasmic vesicles in these antigen presenting cells.

3 The efficient activation of lymphocytes requires adhesive interactions between surface molecules in addition to those involved in antigen recognition. In particular, CD28–CD80 interactions are involved in T cell activation and CD40–CD40L interactions in B cell activation.

4 Mature lymphocytes are found mainly in secondary lymphoid tissues, consisting of the spleen, lymph nodes and MALT.

5 Lymphocytes recirculate between blood, body tissues and secondary lymphoid tissues. The homing of different lymphocytes to different lymphoid tissues is determined by adhesive interactions with high endothelial cells.

6 T cells interact with antigen on presenting cells in the T-dependent areas of secondary lymphoid tissues. B cells activated by these T cells then form germinal centres in the lymphoid follicles where they undergo proliferation, selection and maturation to become plasma cells and memory cells.

7 Immune responses can be down-regulated by a variety of mechanisms. This is necessary for economy, to allow for responses to other antigens, and to avoid excessive tissue damage.

8 Lymphocytes and their subpopulations can be identified and isolated by virtue of their cell surface differentiation molecules. The stimulation of specific lymphocytes by antigen results in measurable activities, e.g. proliferation, cytotoxicity and antibody production.

Further reading

Clark E.A. & Ledbetter J.A. (1994) How B and T cells talk to each other. *Nature*, **367**, 425–428.

Hogg N. & Landis R.C. (1993) Adhesion molecules in cell interactions. *Current Opinion in Immunology*, **5**, 383–390.

Janeway C.A. (1994) How the immune system recognizes invaders. In *Life, Death and the Immune System: Scientific American: A Special Issue*. W.H. Freeman, New York.

Jenkins M.K. & Johnson J.G. (1993) Molecules involved in T-cell costimulation. *Current*

Opinion in Immunology, **5**, 361–367.

Knight S.C. & Stagg A.J. (1993) Antigen-presenting cell types. *Current Opinion in Immunology*, **5**, 374–382.

Liu Y.-J., Johnson G.D., Gordon J. & MacLennan I.C.M. (1992) Germinal centres in T-cell-dependent antibody responses. *Immunology Today*, **13**, 17–21.

MacLennan I.C.M. (1993) The structure and function of secondary lymphoid tissues. In Lachmann P.J., Peters D.K., Rosen F.S. & Walport M.J. eds, *Clinical Aspects of Immunology*, 5th edn. Blackwell Scientific Publications, Oxford.

Neefjes J.J. & Momburg F. (1993) Cell biology of antigen presentation. *Current Opinion in Immunology*, **5**, 27–34.

Parker D.C. (1993) B lymphocytes and B lymphocyte activation. In Lachmann P.J., Peters D.K., Rosen F.S. & Walport M.J. eds, *Clinical Aspects of Immunology*, 5th edn. Blackwell Scientific Publications, Oxford.

Picker L.J. (1994) Control of lymphocyte homing. *Current Opinion in Immunology*, **6**, 394–406.

Stout R.D. (1993) Macrophage activation by T cells: cognate and non-cognate signals. *Current Opinion in Immunology*, **5**, 398–403.

Terhorst C. & Regueiro J.R. (1993) T cell activation. In Lachmann P.J., Peters D.K., Rosen F.S. & Walport M.J. eds, *Clinical Aspects of Immunology*, 5th edn. Blackwell Scientific Publications, Oxford.

CHAPTER 5

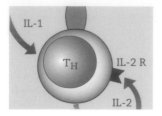

Cytokines

An array of regulatory proteins produced and secreted by lymphocytes and other cells are required to coordinate immune activity. Such molecules produced by lymphocytes are termed **lymphokines**, while those derived from monocytes/macrophages are termed **monokines**. They belong to the general category of **cytokines**, which have a wide range of biological functions extending beyond the immune system. Initially, cytokines were given names relating to their functions. This led to confusion since a single cytokine can have various activities: for example, 'lymphocyte-activating factor' and 'endogenous pyrogen' turned out to be the same molecule, which is now known as interleukin-1. The term **interleukin** (IL) was introduced as part of a classification of agreed names for particular cytokines. In order for a regulatory molecule to qualify for a particular interleukin designation, its gene must have been cloned and sequenced, and shown to be different from previously described molecules.

Table 5.1 indicates the variety of defined cytokines with immune functions. They are all proteins (which are often glycosylated) and have various roles in regulating the amplitude and duration of immune and inflammatory responses. Cytokines are usually produced transiently, exert their effects at very low concentrations and act on cells within close range of the cells from which they are secreted. They mediate their actions by binding to specific cell surface receptors, leading to changes in gene expression which modify cell behaviour. Extensive experimentation has resulted in a bewildering number of cellular effects being attributed to various cytokines both within the immune system and in other contexts. Here we describe four general areas of immune activity in which they are of particular importance.

CYTOKINES: SOURCES AND FUNCTIONS

Cytokine	Immune cells	Other cells	Immunological effects
IL-1α,β	Monocytes/ macrophages	Endothelial, epithelial and neuronal cells, fibroblasts	Activation of T and B cells, macrophages and endothelium. Stimulation of acute phase response
IL-2	T cells		Proliferation and/or activation of T, B and LGL
IL-3	T cells, mast cells, thymic epithelium	Keratinocytes, neuronal cells	Proliferation of pluripotent stem cells. Production of various blood cell types
IL-4	T and B cells, macrophages, mast cells and basophils, bone marrow stroma	–	Activation of B cells. Differentiation of $T_H 2$ cells and suppression of $T_H 1$ cells
IL-5	T cells, mast cells	–	Development, activation and chemoattraction of eosinophils
IL-6	T cells, monocytes or macrophages	Fibroblasts, hepatocytes, endothelial and neuronal cells	Activation of haemopoietic stem cells. Differentiation of B and T cells. Production of acute phase proteins
IL-7	Bone marrow stroma	–	Growth of B cell precursors. Proliferation and cytotoxic activity of T cells
IL-8	T cells, monocytes, neutrophils	Endothelial and epithelial cells, fibroblasts	Chemoattraction of neutrophils, T cells, basophils. Activation of neutrophils
IL-9	T cells	–	Development of erythroid precursors
IL-10	T and B cells, macrophages	Keratinocytes	Suppression of macrophage functions and $T_H 1$ cells. Activation of B cells
IL-11	Bone marrow stroma	Trophoblasts	Stimulation of haemopoietic precursors. Production of acute phase proteins
IL-12	B cells, macrophages	–	Differentiation of $T_H 1$ cells. Activation of LGL and T cells
IL-13	T cells	–	Activation of B cells. Inhibition of monocytes or macrophages
IL-14	T cells	–	Proliferation of activated B cells but inhibition of immunoglobulin secretion

Continued on p. 70

Table 5.1 Cytokines and their immunological functions.

CYTOKINES: SOURCES AND FUNCTIONS

Cytokine	Immune cells	Other cells	Immunological effects
IL-15	T cells	–	Proliferation of T cells
TNF-α	Macrophages, lymphocytes, neutrophils	Astrocytes, endothelium, smooth muscle	Activation of macrophages, granulocytes, cytotoxic cells and endothelium. Enhanced HLA class I expression. Stimulation of acute phase response. Antitumour effects
TNF-β	T cells	–	Similar to TNF-α
IFN-α,β	T and B cells, monocyte or macrophages	Fibroblasts	Antiviral activity. Stimulation of macrophages and LGL. Enhanced HLA class I expression
IFN-γ	T and LGL	–	Antiviral activity. Stimulation of macrophages and endothelium. Enhanced HLA class I and class II expression. Suppression of T_H2 cells
G-CSF	T cells, macrophages, neutrophils	Fibroblasts, endothelium	Development and activation of neutrophils
M-CSF	T cells, macrophages, neutrophils	Fibroblasts, endothelium	Development and activation of monocytes/macrophages
GM-CSF	T cells, macrophages, mast cells, neutrophils, eosinophils	Fibroblasts, endothelium	Differentiation of pluripotent stem cells. Development of neutrophils, eosinophils and macrophages
TGF-β	T cells, monocytes	Chondrocytes, osteoblasts, osteoclasts, platelets, fibroblasts	Inhibition of T and B cell proliferation and LGL activity

IL, interleukin; TNF, tumour necrosis factor; IFN, interferon; CSF, colony stimulating factor; TGF, transforming growth factor.

Table 5.1 (continued)

Functions of immunological cytokines

ACTIVATION OF CELLS OF THE IMMUNE SYSTEM

The actions of cytokines, in addition to direct cellular interactions, are necessary for the stimulation of T and B lymphocytes. As well as presenting antigen to T_H cells, antigen presenting cells (APC) secrete IL-1 which enhances T cell activation (Fig 5 1) Following this initial stimulation, the T_H cell secretes IL-2 and starts to express high-affinity receptors for this interleukin. The binding of IL-2 to these receptors on the same T cell then stimulates its proliferation. Interleukin-2 and other cytokines produced by activated T cells stimulate activity in various other cells of the immune system. For example, IL-2 stimulates cytotoxic T cells and natural killer cells, and interferon-γ activates macrophages. The interferons also stimulate HLA expression, thereby enhancing antigen presentation.

Several cytokines contribute to B cell activation, replication and differentiation into plasma cells: these include IL-4 and IL-6, as illustrated in Fig. 5.2. Furthermore, some cytokines stimulate B cells to switch from IgM to the synthesis of other isotypes of antibodies: e.g. IL-4 promotes the production of IgG4 and IgE.

T_H1 VERSUS T_H2 CELLS

Recent evidence indicates that T_H cells vary in their ability to produce the

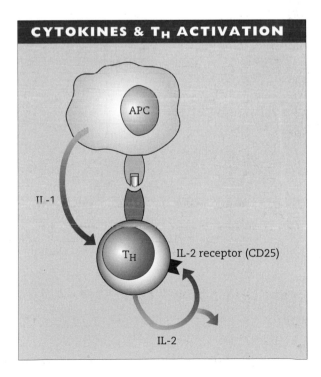

CYTOKINES & T_H ACTIVATION

Fig. 5.1 The role of cytokines in T helper (T_H) cell activation. In response to IL-2, the activated T cell starts to divide and produces other cytokines. APC, antigen presenting cell.

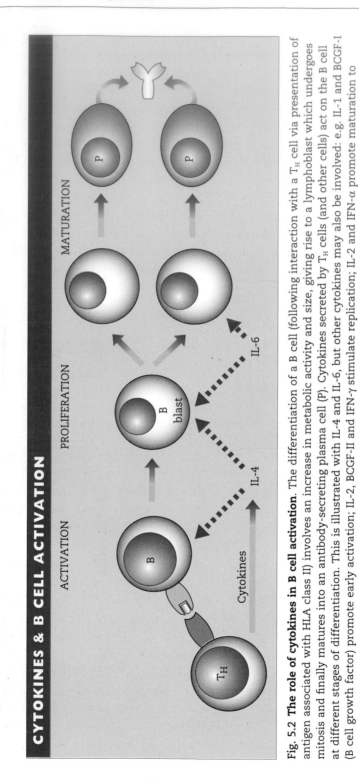

CYTOKINES & B CELL ACTIVATION

Fig. 5.2 **The role of cytokines in B cell activation**. The differentiation of a B cell (following interaction with a T_H cell via presentation of antigen associated with HLA class II) involves an increase in metabolic activity and size, giving rise to a lymphoblast which undergoes mitosis and finally matures into an antibody-secreting plasma cell (P). Cytokines secreted by T_H cells (and other cells) act on the B cell at different stages of differentiation. This is illustrated with IL-4 and IL-6, but other cytokines may also be involved: e.g. IL-1 and BCGF-I (B cell growth factor) promote early activation; IL-2, BCGF-II and IFN-γ stimulate replication; IL-2 and IFN-α promote maturation to plasma cells.

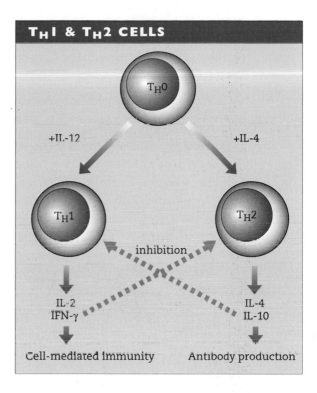

Fig. 5.3 The contrasting roles of T_H1 and T_H2 cells.

combinations of cytokines which preferentially stimulate either cell-mediated or antibody-mediated immunity. As illustrated in Fig. 5.3, **T_H1 cells** produce, amongst other cytokines, IL-2 and IFN-γ which stimulate cytotoxic cells and macrophages leading to cell-mediated immunity. By contrast, **T_H2 cells** produce IL-4 and IL-10 which stimulate B cells and antibody production. These two subsets of helper cells are thought to arise from a common precursor designated T_H0. Macrophage-derived IL-12 stimulates T_H1 development whereas IL-4 (possibly from mast cells or basophils) stimulates the development of T_H2 cells. T_H1 and T_H2 cells are mutually inhibitory through the cytokines they produce: IFN-γ inhibits the proliferation of T_H2 cells whereas IL-10 (and, to some extent, IL-4) inhibits the development and activity of T_H1 cells.

A bias towards activation of T_H1 or T_H2 cells can influence the effectiveness of the immune response against different infectious pathogens. As discussed in Chapter 11, protection against microbes which infect cells usually requires cell-mediated responses whereas extracellular pathogens are most often eliminated by antibody-dependent mechanisms.

This is illustrated in Table 5.2 for *Mycobacterium leprae* which can infect macrophages where it survives and grows in cytoplasmic vesicles. The predominance of T_H1 or T_H2 activity in the immune response then influences whether tuberculoid or lepromatous leprosy results.

HAEMOPOIESIS

A number of cytokines direct the proliferation and differentiation of leucocyte progenitors in the bone marrow. There are specific colony-stimulating factors for macrophage and granulocyte lineages (M-CSF and G-CSF, respectively) and eosinophil differentiation is stimulated by IL-5. Interleukin-3 and GM-CSF stimulate stem cells (from which all blood cell lineages are derived), as well as cooperating with other cytokines in the development of the different lineages.

INFLAMMATION

Many cytokines contribute to the inflammatory process by activating lymphocytes and other leucocytes. In addition, IL-1, IFN-γ and tumour necrosis factor-α (TNF-α) induce the expression of adhesion molecules on endothelial cells causing leucocytes in the circulation to adhere to the endothelium at sites of infection or tissue injury (discussed in Chapter 11). The leucocytes then migrate into tissues by a process called

CYTOKINES AND DISEASE

Event	Development of tuberculoid leprosy	Development of lepromatous leprosy
T_H activation: cytokine production	Activation of T_H1: production of IFN-γ	Activation of T_H2: production of IL-4
Effector cell stimulation: effects on mycobacteria	Activation of macrophages: intracellular digestion of mycobacteria in cytoplasmic vesicles	Activation of B cells: antibodies have no access to intracellular mycobacteria
Resulting pathology	Some inflammatory tissue damage, but destruction of mycobacteria	Growth of mycobacteria and severe tissue damage

Table 5.2 The influence of cytokine production on disease pathogenesis following infection of macrophages by *Mycobacterium leprae*.

chemotaxis in which they respond to a variety of chemical attractants emanating from the site of infection or injury. Interleukin-8 is one member of a large family of chemotactic peptides called **chemokines**. Different members of this family preferentially attract neutrophils, monocytes or T cells.

The systemic response to infection or injury, affecting tissues throughout the body, is termed the **acute phase response**. The cytokines IL-1, IL-6 and TNF-α stimulate these effects by acting on a variety of cell types: this is discussed further in Chapter 11.

CYTOSTATIC, CYTOTOXIC AND ANTIVIRAL ACTIVITIES

The ability to inhibit cellular proliferation or induce cell death, especially of certain tumour cell types, is associated with particular cytokines. The closely related molecules TNF-α and TNF-β show these activities, as do the interferons (α, β and γ). Tumour necrosis factor derives its name from the ability to stimulate tumour necrosis and regression *in vivo*, while the interferons are so named because they interfere with (i.e. inhibit) viral replication in infected cells and have a defensive role in the early stages of viral infection. IFN-α and IFN-β are closely related to each other and can be produced by various cells. IFN-γ is structurally unrelated to IFN-α and IFN-β, and is produced by activated T cells and natural killer cells.

The cytokine network

It is important to realize that not all the effects of cytokines that have been elucidated by experimentation *in vitro* may be synonymous with their actions *in vivo*: physiological activity may be affected by local concentration, stability and distribution within tissues. Each cytokine cannot be considered in isolation but should be regarded as part of a network of interacting mediators. Firstly, in many instances cytokines are interdependent in mediating maximal effects: this can be because different cytokines are required for each stage of a multistep process (as in the activation, proliferation and differentiation of B cells), or because particular combinations of cytokines are synergistic (e.g. IFN-γ and TNF-α in antiviral, antiproliferative and HLA-inducing activities). Secondly, particular cytokines may induce the production of other mediators and/or their receptors (e.g. IFN-γ induces synthesis of TNF-α and expression of cell surface receptors for TNF-α). Thirdly, some cytokines may inhibit the action of others.

Cytokines and therapy

An understanding of the potent biological effects of cytokines coupled with their large-scale production by the biotechnology industry has led to their application as therapeutic agents. For example, the immuno-stimulatory effects of IL-2 and IFN-γ have been used to boost beneficial immune responses; colony stimulating factors to promote haemopoiesis, and IFN-α as an antitumour or antiviral agent. Conversely, some autoimmune and inflammatory conditions are characterized by excessive cytokine activity which can be inhibited therapeutically. For example, TNF-α has been found to perpetuate inflammatory joint damage in rheumatoid arthritis, and inhibition of this cytokine is beneficial in patients with this disease.

KEY POINTS

1 Cytokines are proteins secreted by various cell types and regulate the amplitude and duration of immune and inflammatory responses.
2 The immunological functions of cytokines include regulating the activity of cells of the immune system, promoting haemopoiesis, inflammatory effects, and cytostatic, cytotoxic and antiviral activities.
3 The immunological effects of particular cells is influenced by the profile of cytokines they produce. For example, T_H1 and T_H2 cells promote cell-mediated and antibody-mediated immunity, respectively.
4 Interaction between the cellular effects of different cytokines, either to enhance or inhibit each others' actions, determines the overall biological effect.
5 The beneficial or detrimental effects of cytokines in disease situations can be manipulated for therapeutic benefit.

Further reading

Burke F., Naylor M.S., Davies B. & Balkwill F. (1993) The cytokine wallchart. *Immunology Today*, **14**, 165–170.
O'Garra A. & Murphy K. (1994) Role of cytokines in determining T-lymphocyte function. *Current Opinion in Immunology*, **6**, 458–466.
Paul W.E. & Seder R.A. (1994) Lymphocyte responses and cytokines. *Cell*, **76**, 241–251.
Schall T.J. & Bacon K.B. (1994) Chemokines, leukocyte trafficking, and inflammation. *Current Opinion in Immunology*, **6**, 865–873.

CHAPTER 6

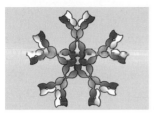

Immunoglobulins

All vertebrates possess immunoglobulin-like molecules. They are synthesized and secreted by end cells of the B cell lineage, i.e. plasma cells. These serum proteins were first discovered a century ago by Paul Ehrlich and his colleagues by virtue of their ability to confer protection, i.e. immunity, against a number of important bacterial infections. Their function as antigen-recognition molecules gave rise to the alternative term, antibodies. They are largely confined to the broad and heterogeneous band of γ-globulins observed on electrophoresis (Fig. 6.1) and show considerable diversity of structure and function.

Structure

The typical immunoglobulin molecule is asymmetrically composed of four polypeptide chains linked by disulphide bridges (Fig. 6.2). The larger chains are designated **heavy** and the smaller **light**: it is the combined amino-terminal ends of these two chains which create the two antigen combining sites of the molecule. Within a given immunoglobulin molecule the heavy chains are identical with each other, as are the light chains, so that the two antigen-combining sites have the same specificity for antigen. The carboxy-terminal portions of the heavy chains trigger various effector functions following combination of the immunoglobulin molecule with its specific antigen. Several immunoglobulin fragments can be prepared using proteolytic enzymes and these have been of value in unravelling the functional activities of different parts of these molecules. Digestion with papain cleaves on the amino-terminal side of the inter-heavy chain disulphide bonds, yielding two **Fab** fragments, thus designated because they retain the ability to recognize antigen (i.e. **F**ragment antigen-binding). The other fragment can be readily crystallized and was thus termed

77

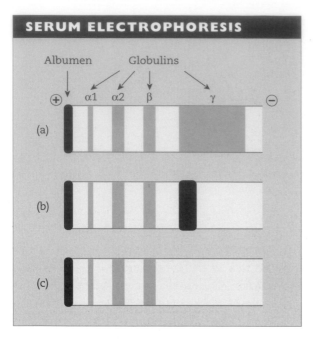

Fig. 6.1 Protein electrophoresis of (a) normal serum, (b) serum showing a compact band of monoclonal immunoglobulin (from a case of myeloma) and (c) serum from a patient with hypogammaglobulinaemia.

Fc (i.e. **F**ragment **c**rystallizable). Pepsin digestion cleaves the molecule to the carboxy-terminal side of the inter-heavy chain disulphide bonds and this generates a Fab dimer designated $F(ab')_2$, leaving a rather smaller Fc fragment designated pFc'.

VARIABLE AND CONSTANT DOMAINS

Figure 6.3 illustrates the immunoglobulin molecule in a Y configuration and emphasizes the flexible hinge region which permits considerable movement of the Fab arms. Both light and heavy polypeptide chains consist of a series of similar globular subunits or **domains**. Each domain consists of a stretch of about 110 amino acids of polypeptide chain folded into two layers of β-pleated sheet held together by a single intrachain disulphide bridge giving a roughly cylindrical conformation. Although there is considerable overall similarity between the various light and heavy chain domains, the amino-terminal domain shows a marked degree of variation of many of its amino acid residues and is termed **variable** in contrast to the other domains which vary comparatively little from each other and are termed **constant**. Light chains contain one variable and one constant domain (V_L and C_L) whereas heavy chains contain one variable domain (V_H) and three or four constant domains (C_H1, C_H2, C_H3

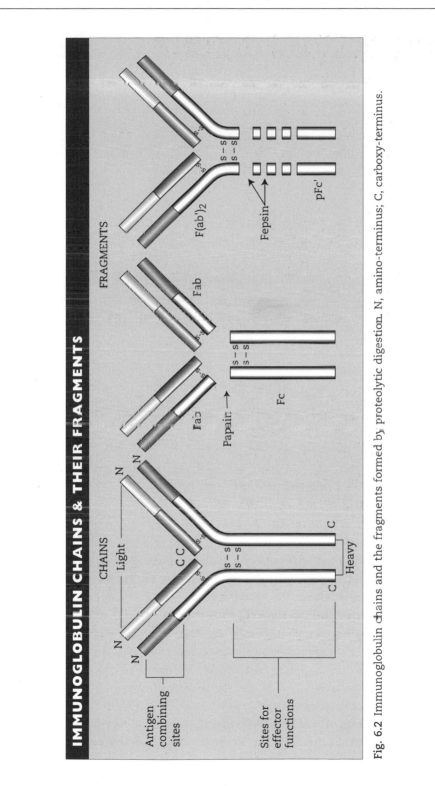

Fig. 6.2 Immunoglobulin chains and the fragments formed by proteolytic digestion. N, amino-terminus; C, carboxy-terminus.

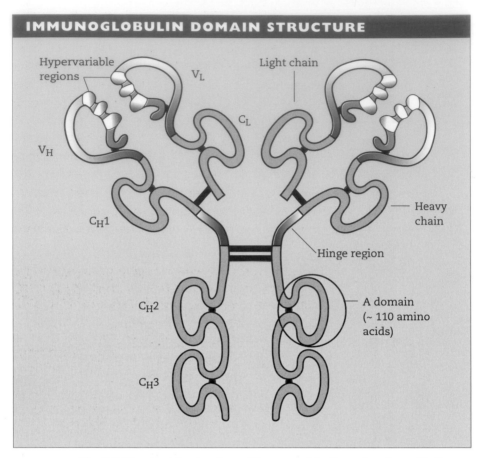

IMMUNOGLOBULIN DOMAIN STRUCTURE

Hypervariable regions

V_L

Light chain

C_L

V_H

C_H1

Heavy chain

Hinge region

C_H2

A domain (~ 110 amino acids)

C_H3

Fig. 6.3 The domain structure of immunoglobulin molecules, with the domains shown as peptide loops.

and C_H4) depending on the class of immunoglobulin. The domain structure of immunoglobulins is very similar to the pattern of polypeptide looping found in T cell receptors as well as that seen in both kinds of HLA glycoprotein and other cell surface adhesion molecules (see Fig. 2.3). This suggests that they have all developed as specializations of an ancestral recognition molecule present upon the surface of most kinds of cell. They are together regarded as members of the **immunoglobulin superfamily**.

THE ANTIGEN-COMBINING SITE

Much of the variation found between immunoglobulins of different antigenic specificities is located within three 'hot spots' or **hyper-variable regions** (HVR-1, -2 and -3) (Fig. 6.3) which lie in close proximity to each other within the folded structure of the variable domain. Thus, the most variable parts of this domain are brought together to form the **antigen-combining site** or cleft consisting of the three hypervariable regions from the light chain and a further three from the adjacent heavy chain (Fig. 6.4a).

The specific chemistry and shape of this combining site is complementary to the specific chemistry and shape of the **antigenic determinant** or **epitope** (Fig. 6.4b & Chapter 2) thus, the HVR lining the combining site are also referred to as **complementarity determining regions**. The term 'combining site' is confined to that part of the molecule which specifically interacts with the epitope, whereas the entire area of surface

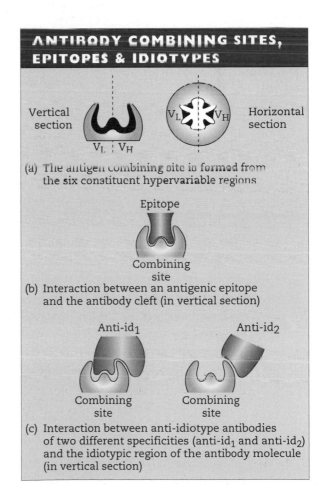

Fig. 6.4 Spatial configuration of the antigen-combining site or cleft and its interaction with epitopes and anti-idiotypes.

conformation which is unique to an immunoglobulin molecule of particular antigenic specificity is known as the **idiotype** (from the Greek *idios*, meaning 'private'). These unique shapes and surfaces can themselves be recognized by other antibodies which are then referred to as having **anti-idiotype** specificity (Fig. 6.4c). If they interact sufficiently with the antigen-combining site, they may block the combination of antigen epitope with it (e.g. anti-id$_1$) or, if they react with a more peripheral part, they may not inhibit epitope combination (e.g. anti-id$_2$).

AFFINITY AND AVIDITY

The strength of binding or association of a single epitope for a single combining site in a homogeneous system is termed **affinity**. The more usual situation whereby an antigen bearing several epitopes combines with a variety of specific antibody molecules, each with their own combining sites, is a very heterogeneous system and the term **avidity** is used to indicate the average strength of this association. The former is as easy to measure as the strength of binding of a hormone for its receptor: the latter is a much more complicated affair. Avidity also refers to the combined affinities of the two (or more) antigen-combining sites of a single antibody molecule, as illustrated in Fig. 6.5. The number of combining sites defines the **valency** of the antibody (e.g. two for IgG, ten for IgM), and the equivalent valency of the antigen is the number of repeats of the particular epitope it carries.

Classes and subclasses

There are five classes of immunoglobulin in man: IgG, IgA, IgM, IgD and IgE (Table 6.1 & Fig. 6.6). These show important structural and functional differences within the constant regions of their heavy chains and, in the case of IgG and IgA, subdivide further into subclasses. Each of these structural variants is present in all normal individuals. They can be

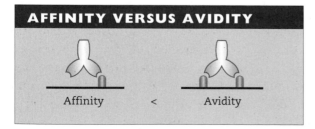

Fig. 6.5 A comparison of the affinity and avidity of binding of a monomeric antibody molecule.

CHARACTERISTICS OF IMMUNOGLOBULINS

	IgG	IgA	IgM	IgD	IgE
Physical properties					
Molecular weight	150 000	160 000 (monomer)	900 000	180 000	190 000
Number of four-chain units	1	1 or 2	5	1	1
Heavy chains	γ	α	μ	δ	ε
Light chains	κ or λ	κ or λ	κ or λ	κ or λ	κ or λ
Other peptide chains	–	J* ± S†	J*	–	–
Subclasses	γ1 γ2 γ3 γ4	α1 α2	–	–	–
Serum concentration (g l⁻¹)	c. 10 (65% 25% 6% 4%)	c. 2 (85% 15%)	c. 1	c. 0.03	c. 0.0002 (i.e. 200 ng ml⁻¹)
Biological activities					
Complement fixation:					
Classical pathway	γ1 γ2 γ3		++	–	–
Alternative pathway	+**	+	–	–	–
Phagocyte binding	γ1 γ3	+§	–	–	+§
Mast cell binding	–	–	–	–	++
LGL binding	γ1 γ3	–	–	–	–
Eosinophil binding	γ1 γ3 γ4	–	–	–	+
Extravascular diffusion	γ1 γ2 γ3 γ4	+	–	–	+
Mucosal transfer		++	+	–	–
Placental transfer	γ1 γ2 γ3 γ4	–	–	–	–

* J, J chain; † S, secretory piece; ** see text; § see Table 8.2.

Table 6.1 Physical and biological characteristics of immunoglobulins.

identified and quantified by specific antisera raised in another species and are referred to as **isotypes**. Other, single amino acid, variations occur as heritable polymorphisms and are known as **allotypes**. These have been identified within IgG (the Gm system), IgA (the Am system) and on K chains (the Km system).

Each class (or subclass) of immunoglobulin consists of four-chain units as depicted in Figs 6.3 and 6.6. In IgG, IgD and IgE, these are monomeric whereas IgA often occurs as a dimer and IgM almost always as a pentamer. The heavy chains of each class are given the equivalent Greek letter, e.g. γ for IgG (see Table 6.1). The light chains can be of two types, kappa (κ) or lambda (λ) and the two light chains of a single immunoglobulin molecule are of the same type, i.e. *either* κ or λ. Both

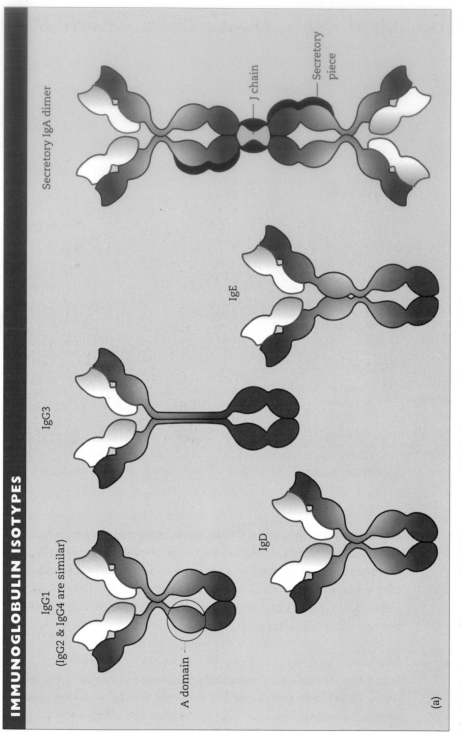

Fig. 6.6 Structure of immunoglobulin isotypes, with the domains shown as globular units.

IMMUNOGLOBULIN ISOTYPES

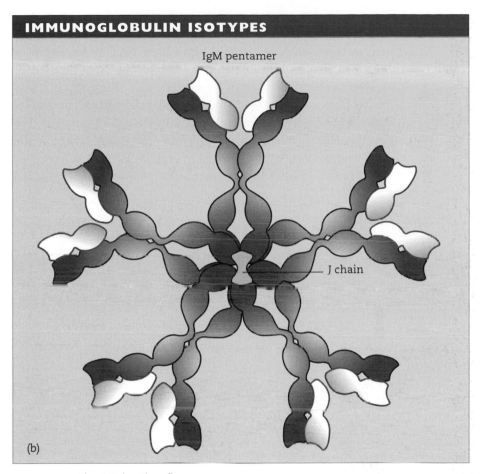

Fig. 6.6 (continued)

polymeric forms (IgA and IgM) contain an additional peptide known as **J chain** (15000 daltons molecular weight) which plays a part in holding the monomeric subunits together. Dimeric IgA, present in secretions, contains a further component known as **secretory piece** (70000 daltons molecular weight) which is derived from cells of the secretory epithelium through which IgA is transported.

IgG

This is the most plentiful immunoglobulin in internal body fluids and is produced particularly during secondary immune responses. The γ chains contain three constant regions (Cγ1, Cγ2 and Cγ3) which are involved in the different effector functions of the molecule (Table 6.1). The three most plentiful subclasses (IgG1, IgG2 and IgG3) activate the classical complement pathway via the Cγ2 domain (see Table 6.2 and Chapter 7). IgG in aggregated form can enhance existing activation of the alternative complement pathway but the particular involvement of individual subclasses and domains is unclear.

The subclasses IgG1 and IgG3 (and, to some extent, IgG4) also interact with three Fc receptors expressed on various cell types (Table 6.2). The high affinity FcγRI and FcγRII bind in the lower hinge region close to the Cγ2 domain, whereas both Cγ2 and Cγ3 may be involved in binding to FcγRIII. The interaction of microbe-associated IgG with macrophages and

Fc BINDING PROTEINS

Immunoglobulin binding protein	Immunoglobulin isotypes bound	Domains involved	Sites of binding protein expression
Fc$_\gamma$RI*	IgG (1 = 3 > 4)	Cγ2/hinge	Macrophages, neutrophils
Fc$_\gamma$RII*	IgG (1, 3)	Cγ2/hinge	Macrophages, neutrophils, eosinophils, basophils, B cells, platelets, Langerhans cells
Fc$_\gamma$RIII*	IgG (1, 3)	Cγ3/4†	Macrophages, neutrophils, large granular lymphocytes placental trophoblasts
Fc$_\mu$R	IgM	Cμ3/4†	Some B and T cells
Fc$_\alpha$R*	IgA (1, 2)	Cα2†	Macrophages, neutrophils, eosinophils
Fc$_\varepsilon$RI*	IgE	Cε2–3	Mast cells, basophils
Fc$_\varepsilon$RII	IgE	Cε2, 3, 4	Monocytes, eosinophils, activated B cells, platelets, follicular dendritic cells
Polyimmunoglobulin receptor*	Dimeric IgA	Unknown	Mucosal epithelium
C1q	IgG (1, 2, 3) IgM	Cγ2 Cμ3	Plasma and tissue fluid
Protein A	IgG (1, 2, 4)	Cγ2–3	*Staphylococcus aureus*
Protein G	IgG (1–4)		*Staphylococcus aureus*

* Members of the immunoglobulin superfamily.
† The binding site within the Fc region has not been precisely identified.

Table 6.2 Proteins which bind to the Fc region of immunoglobulins.

neutrophils facilitates the phagocytosis and killing of the bound microbe (Chapter 8), while IgG interacting with the surfaces of eosinophils (Chapter 9) and large granular lymphocytes (Chapter 10) facilitates the lysis of extracellular targets. The bacterium *Staphylococcus aureus* produces Fc binding proteins (protein A and protein G) which, by inhibiting the Fc-dependent functions of IgG, may aid bacterial survival (and see Chapter 11).

All four subclasses of IgG interact with Fc receptors in the placenta and are transported into the fetal circulation.

IgA

This is the major immunoglobulin of external secretions. It is particularly evident during the secondary immune response to antigen gaining access via mucosal surfaces. It does not activate complement by the classical pathway but is able to stabilize the alternative pathway C3 convertase (see Chapter 7). It also has an affinity for phagocyte surfaces although this is less than that of IgG1 and IgG3. Much of its protective value may be due to its direct combination with and neutralization of pathogenic micro-organisms in the gut and respiratory tract without necessarily involving any other effector systems.

IgA dimers and their associated **J chains** are produced by submucosal plasma cells. They gain access to the lumen of the gut and other mucosal sites by complexing with a receptor for polymeric immunoglobulin present on the surface of enterocytes and hepatocytes. This receptor has a high affinity for J chain and, after combination with it, dimeric IgA is transported across the cell by endocytosis and then released with the outer portion of the poly-Ig receptor still attached. This component is designated **secretory piece**: and may protect secretory IgA from proteolytic cleavage.

Dimeric, J chain-containing, IgA also gains access to the portal circulation and is transported into bile via the poly-Ig receptor present on hepatocytes. As most circulating IgA in man (in contrast to mice and rats) is present in monomeric form it is unlikely that this is an important route for the transport of secretory IgA into the gut under normal conditions.

IgM

This is the key immunoglobulin of the primary response and is a large pentameric molecule containing 10 antigen-combining sites, giving the potential for high avidity binding to antigen. The five monomeric units are linked together with a single J chain molecule. Its heavy (μ) chains have four constant domains (Fig. 6.6). IgM is an efficient activator of the classical complement pathway (Table 6.1). The level of specific antibody belonging to this class fades with progressive exposure to specific antigen in favour of other isotypes, e.g. IgG and IgA. T cells are thought to have a role in governing the mechanism of isotype switching, and the nature of the immunoglobulin gene arrangements which mediate this event are described below. Owing to its relatively large size, IgM does not normally escape from the circulation into tissue fluids. However, J chain-containing IgM has an affinity for the poly-Ig receptor and when there is a relative dearth of IgA, as in IgA deficiency, then IgM can appear in secretions linked to secretory piece.

IgD

This is normally present in minute concentrations in blood and other body fluids but is readily detected on the surface of many early B cells in conjunction with IgM. It is thought not to mediate any of the usual effector functions attributed to other immunoglobulins but may have a role as antigen receptor on early B cells.

IgE

This monomeric immunoglobulin has four constant domains (like IgM) and, although it is the least plentiful of all immunoglobulins, its presence can be dramatically felt by its ability to bind to high-affinity Fc receptors ($Fc_\varepsilon RI$) on the surface of mast cells and basophils (Tables 6.1 & 6.2) and, when complexed with specific antigen, to trigger the release of inflammatory mediators (see Chapter 9). Its physiological role may be to function with mast cells as a 'gatekeeper' regulating the exit of cells and plasma into extravascular sites. Certain other cell types express a lower affinity receptor for IgE ($Fc_\varepsilon RII$): IgE binding to these receptors on eosinophils may be important in immunity to parasitic worms.

Triggering of effector systems

In some situations antibodies can act alone, e.g. neutralization of bacterial toxins and viruses, and inhibition of flagellar motility. However, their effect is most striking when they are able to trigger and recruit the assistance of other effector molecules and cells, e.g. complement and phagocytes (Tables 1.2 & 6.1). Clearly, it would be inappropriate for this event to be mediated by uncomplexed immunoglobulin and strict requirements have to be fulfilled before the appropriate signal is generated. For activation of the classical complement pathway by IgG, two adjacent IgG molecules have to be stabilized within an immune complex or IgG aggregate and at an appropriate distance from each other such that a minimum of two of the six heads of the first complement protein (C1q) can interact with the Cγ2 domain which then causes a steric rearrangement of the C1 complex with activation of C1r and C1s (see Chapter 7). Each of the other domains in the IgG molecule is stabilized by a hydrophobic interaction with its homologous partner whereas the Cγ2 domains are partly masked by carbohydrate and protrude outward, facilitating their interaction with C1q. A single IgM molecule, with five Fc regions, can interact with C1q by itself. However, this again only occurs when the antibody is complexed with antigen, which is thought to distort the molecule so as to expose the Fc binding sites for C1q within the Cμ3 domains.

Each of the other effector functions, e.g. phagocyte activation and mast cell degranulation, is also triggered by the approximation and stabilization of Fc domains within complexed antibody. The requirement for cross-linking of surface IgE on the mast cell has been shown by the demonstration that mast cell degranulation can be produced by intact divalent anti-IgE but not with monovalent Fab fragments.

Immunoglobulin genes

It was a source of puzzlement for many years how, if each protein (or polypeptide chain) is encoded by a single gene, immunoglobulin molecules with identical constant regions but a vast repertoire of different variable domains could be synthesized. The discovery of non-expressed intervening sequences or **introns**, as well as peptide coding sequences or **exons** within chromosomal DNA, and the realization that rearrangements of these sequences were possible have helped to clarify this problem.

It was difficult to comprehend how up to 10^8 different antibody specificities could be encoded by genes inherited in the germline but it is now clear that many of the rearrangements of DNA and RNA that take place during B cell differentiation make significant contributions to the total diversity of the antibody molecules which are produced. Figure 6.7 illustrates the way in which rearrangements are made in the germline DNA coding for κ light chain proteins. Each variable domain is encoded by two gene segments (i.e. exons): a variable (V) gene segment makes the larger contribution (including HVR1 and HVR2), and a small joining (J) segment. The germline DNA contains about 250 V_κ exons and four expressable J_κ exons on chromosome 2. During B cell development in the bone marrow, random selection for expression of a V_κ and a J_κ exon takes place in each pre-B cell by rearrangement of the DNA to link any

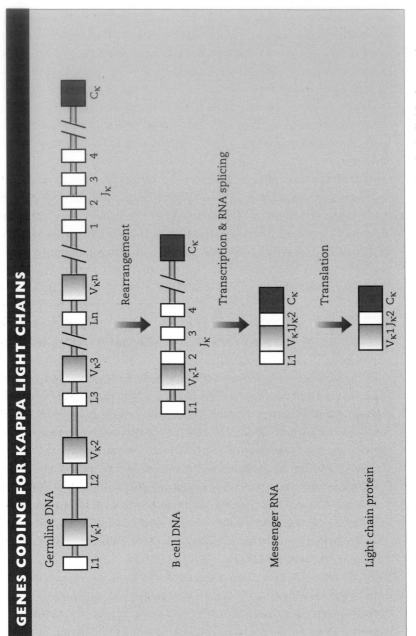

Fig. 6.7 Organization and rearrangement of genes coding for κ light chains. The notation for individual exons is as follows: L, leader; J, joining; $V_\kappa 1 \ldots V_\kappa n$, variable regions; C_κ, constant regions.

one of the V_κ exons with any one of the J_κ exons (e.g. $V_\kappa 1$ and $J_\kappa 2$ in Fig. 6.7). The recombined V–J junction encodes the HVR3 of the variable domain. The single exon for the κ light chain constant domain (C_κ) is located near the J segments (Fig. 6.7). Following transcription of the whole genetic locus into RNA, the RNA between the V–J and C exons is spliced out to yield the uninterrupted V–J–C message which is then translated into the light chain protein (Fig. 6.7).

The λ-light chain locus is on chromosome 22 and the process of rearrangement and expression of the λ genes are very similar to those described above for κ-light chains. However, less diversity of λ variable domains is possible, as there are only three pairs of V_λ and J_λ exons, each linked to a separate C_λ exon.

Further diversity is possible with the rearrangements that take place in the DNA coding for heavy chains on chromosome 14 (Fig. 6.8). As well as a considerable number of V_H exons (between 200 and 1000) and four J_H exons there is an additional group of exons in between, termed the diversity (D) segments. The first step in DNA rearrangement involves the random selection and joining of a D and a J exon, followed by rearrangement to one of the V_H exons. In this case it is the V–D–J junction which forms the heavy chain HVR3. In a naive B cell (i.e. which has not been activated by antigen), RNA splicing joins the transcribed variable domain gene to the C_μ or C_δ constant region RNA to be translated into the heavy chains for IgM and IgD, respectively.

Thus, three genetic elements code for a light chain (V, J and C) and four encode a heavy chain (V, D, J and C), i.e. a total of seven genetic elements encode a complete immunoglobulin protein. Furthermore, within the DNA which encodes each heavy chain constant region, there are separate exons for each C_H domain, i.e. three each for C_δ, C_γ and C_α, and four each for C_μ and C_ε. The genetic mechanism whereby a B cell switches the class of immunoglobulin it produces is described below. The production of both surface and secreted immunoglobulins by a B cell (i.e. antigen receptors and antibodies) is due to the differential expression of an additional exon which encodes the membrane-spanning portion of the surface-bound immunoglobulin.

THE ORIGINS OF DIVERSITY

Several factors contribute to the enormous range of antibody diversity present in higher vertebrates, as listed in Table 6.3. The diversity already encoded within the diploid genome and generated by the random selection of V, D and J exons in each B cell precursor have been considered above. Further diversity within HVR3 is generated during the joining of V

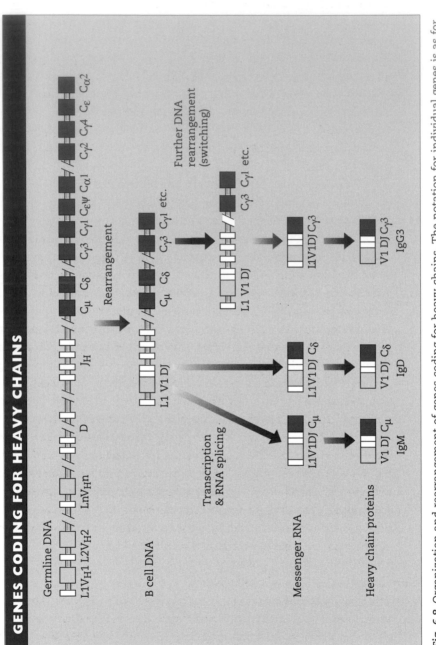

Fig. 6.8 Organization and rearrangement of genes coding for heavy chains. The notation for individual genes is as for Fig. 6.7 with the following addition: D, diversity.

DIVERSITY OF IMMUNOGLOBULIN DOMAINS

Multiple germline genes	Multiple V, D and J exons
Exon rearrangements	Random selection of the V, D and J exons rearranged for expression
Junctional diversity	Imprecise nucleotide alignment and/or insertion of nucleotides at the V–D–J junctions
H–L chain combinations	Independent selection of heavy and light chain variable region genes in each B cell
Somatic mutation	Point mutations in the variable region genes of activated B cells

Table 6.3 Mechanisms which contribute to the diversity of immunoglobulin variable domains.

and J, or V, D and J segments by the random formation of variations in nucleotide sequence at the junctions. These are produced by slight imprecisions of alignment in the DNA sequences being joined and/or the insertion of additional nucleotides. In either case, this can result in the coding of different amino acids at the exon junctions.

The selection and rearrangement of heavy chain V, D and J exons and light chain V and J exons occur independently of one another. This leads to greater binding site diversity since, for example, two B cells expressing identical V_H domains could employ entirely different V_L domains and so have different antigenic specificities.

A final level of diversification occurs in activated proliferating B cells during the course of an immune response. This involves point mutations (i.e. single nucleotide substitutions during DNA replication), particularly within HVR-encoding sequences, which can result in changes in the antigen contact amino acid residues. In some cases this **somatic mutation** produces B cells with receptors of higher affinity for the antigen which are therefore selected in germinal centres for maturation into plasma cells or memory cells (see Chapter 4).

Allelic exclusion and clonal selection

The rearrangement of immunoglobulin genes during B cell development is not always successful, i.e. non-productive arrangements can occur which do not encode functional heavy or light chains. However, each B cell precursor has several opportunities to generate productive rearrangements by virtue of having two alleles of each gene within the diploid genome, together with the possibility of utilizing either type of light chain (i.e. κ or λ). The developmental order of rearrangements starts with each heavy chain allele followed by the κ alleles and finally, if necessary, the λ alleles. A productive rearrangement blocks further rearrangements of a similar type. For example, if one heavy chain allele is successfully rearranged, the other heavy chain allele is never used in that B cell, and a λ chain allele will only be used if both attempts to rearrange the κ chain alleles are non-productive.

This **allelic exclusion** ensures that all the surface and secreted immunoglobulins made by a single B cell have the same V_H and V_L domains and hence the same antigenic specificity. This explains the genetic basis of how an antigen-specific response is mounted by **clonal selection**, as described in Chapter 2. In essence, this means that those lymphocytes bearing receptors that fit the epitope best are preferentially stimulated to divide and produce more cells of the same specificity. It is extremely unusual for only one kind of receptor, i.e. specificity, to be stimulated with the result that a hierarchy of cells is triggered, giving rise to a **polyclonal** response consisting of antibody molecules with a range of affinities for the epitopes concerned. The antibodies produced in a secondary response are likely to be of higher affinity in view of preferential expansion of those clones which best fit the antigen.

Monoclonal or **oligoclonal** responses are usually seen in abnormal situations, e.g. myelomatosis, during recovery following a bone marrow graft or when antibody-producing cells are fused experimentally with plasmacytoma cells to form a monoclonal hybridoma (see p. 99).

ISOTYPE SWITCHING

The heavy chain constant region genes occur in three groups adjacent to the J_H exons on chromosome 14 (Fig. 6.8). C_μ and C_δ are closest to the J segments, and the others occur in two groups of four (although one of the C_ε genes is a non-productive pseudogene). They are likely to have arisen by tandem gene duplication during evolution and the primordial gene cluster probably took the form C_μ/C_δ followed by C_γ, C_ε and C_α. Production of IgM and IgD with the same variable domains involves differential RNA splicing, whereas switching to expression of the same V–D–J combination with any of the other constant region genes (i.e. $C_\gamma 3$ through to $C_\alpha 2$) requires further DNA rearrangements. This is controlled by 'switch' sequences of DNA in the introns adjacent to each constant region gene which enable loops of DNA to be removed and constant region genes for IgG, IgE and IgA to be located in close proximity to the variable region genes (Fig. 6.8). It is not yet clear what causes one switch sequence to have preference over another, although T lymphocytes and/or their cytokines are involved in the process: for example, IL-4 promotes switching to IgE synthesis, and IL-5 to IgA.

T cell receptor genes

The genes which encode the T cell receptor α and β polypeptide chains are similar to the immunoglobulin genes. The variable domains are encoded by V and J exons for the α-chain, and V, D and J exons for the β-chain. Most of the variability is focused at the V–J and V–D–J junctions, which are thought to form the regions of the combining site which interact with the antigenic peptide held in the binding groove of an HLA molecule. Thus, T cell receptor diversity is generated by the same mechanisms which give rise to the diversity of B cell receptors and antibodies, with the exception that somatic mutation does not occur in T cell receptor genes. Further differences from immunoglobulins concern the constant domains of T cell receptors in that there is no isotypic variation and there is no secreted form of T cell receptors lacking the transmembrane domain.

Exploiting the properties of immunoglobulins

Antigens and antibodies do not combine in fixed proportions, i.e. their union is not stoichiometric. This is illustrated in a standard **quantitative precipitation test** (Fig. 6.9) in which increasing concentrations of antigen are added to a series of tubes containing a constant concentration of antibody. A maximum amount of precipitate is formed at an optimum point but antigen–antibody complexes form at other numerical proportions of antigen and antibody. These **immune complexes** vary in their composition: complexes formed near the point of optimal proportions or **equivalence** are largest and tend to form a lattice whereas those formed in antibody excess or antigen excess are smaller and precipitate less readily. This method can be used to determine the amount of antibody present in an antiserum as well as the valency of the antigen.

LABORATORY METHODS

These principles underlie many different kinds of **immunodiffusion** technique in which antigens and antibodies diffuse toward each other through a transparent support medium, e.g. agar, to form lines of precipitation in the equivalence zone (Fig. 6.10). These methods are used to detect and characterize solutions or extracts of antigens or antibodies (e.g. **double diffusion**), to measure the concentration of a particu-

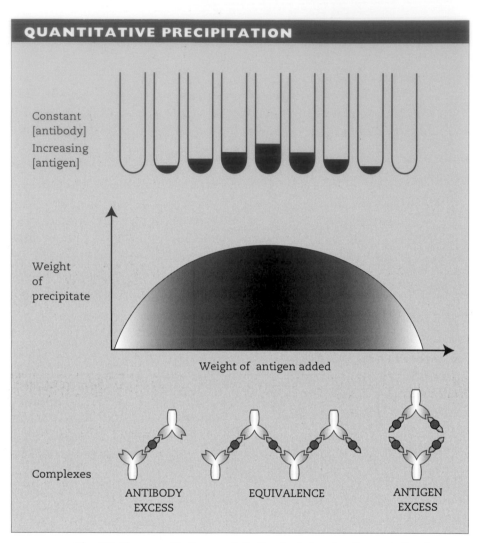

Fig. 6.9 The quantitative precipitation test showing the variation in amount of precipitate formed and the size of complexes at different antigen–antibody ratios.

lar protein antigen (e.g. **radial immunodiffusion**), to detect qualitative differences in proteins present in serum or other fluids (e.g. **immunoelectrophoresis** – and see Fig. 17.2) and to quantify proteins differentially (**two-dimensional immunoelectrophoresis**).

The coupling of antigens to the surface of red cells or other particles provides greater sensitivity for the detection of specific antibodies by **agglutination, lysis** or **complement fixation** (Fig. 6.11). These tech-

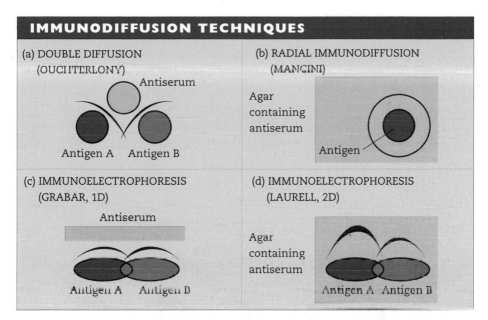

Fig. 6.10 Immunodiffusion techniques for characterizing specific antigens or antibodies.

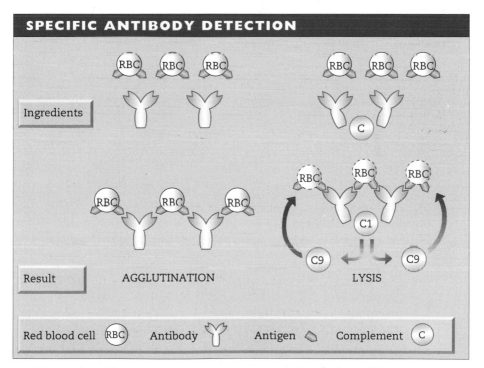

Fig. 6.11 Agglutination and lysis techniques for detecting specific antibodies. Results are often reported as a titre, i.e. the weakest dilution of serum which gives a positive result.

niques still form the mainstay of blood grouping, cross-matching and the detection of many microbial and auto-antibodies.

Immunofluorescence, and techniques using enzyme-labelled (**ELISA**) and radiolabelled (**RIA**) reagents are also widely used to determine the specificity of antigen–antibody reactions (Fig. 6.12) and to examine tissues for the presence of immunological components. Their applications are legion but, as with all laboratory methods, the accuracy and precision of the results obtained depend on the regular use of

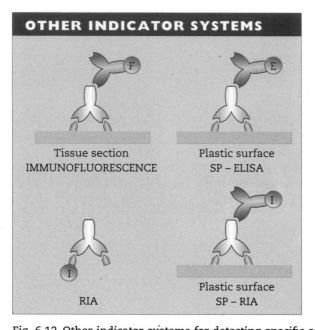

OTHER INDICATOR SYSTEMS

Tissue section
IMMUNOFLUORESCENCE

Plastic surface
SP – ELISA

RIA

Plastic surface
SP – RIA

Fig. 6.12 Other indicator systems for detecting specific antibody. Immunofluorescent techniques involve the reaction of antibody with sections of antigen-containing tissue. After suitable washing, the antibody can be detected using a fluorescein-labelled second antibody (i.e. antiglobulin) and UV microscopy. The solid phase enzyme-linked immunosorbent assay (SP-ELISA) utilizes antigen-coated plastic tubes or wells. Antibody binding is detected using an enzyme-conjugated antiglobulin and the colour generated on addition of substrate is read visually or with a spectrophotometer. Radioimmunoassay (RIA) is used more often to determine amounts of antigen (e.g. hormone) and is a measure of how much a standard amount of radiolabelled antigen is displaced from antibody binding in the presence of the unknown material. Solid-phase RIA is exactly comparable to SP-ELISA except that a radiolabelled antiglobulin is used and the amount of antibody bound is determined by γ counting.

B CELL HYBRIDOMAS MAKE MONOCLONAL ANTIBODIES

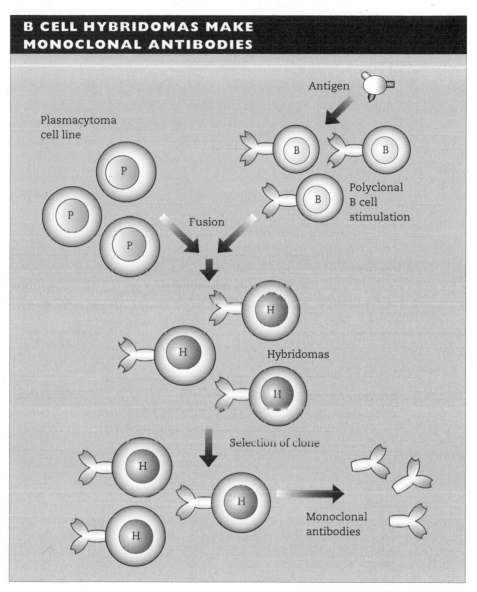

Fig. 6.13 Formation of B cell hybridomas for the production of monoclonal antibodies.

internal and external standards and the rigorous application of quality control protocols.

MONOCLONAL ANTIBODIES FROM HYBRIDOMAS

The production of antibodies by continuously growing **B cell hybridomas** was first described by Köhler and Milstein in 1975.

Monoclonal antibodies derived from hybridoma cell lines are now of great importance in basic and clinical medicine as well as many other areas of biology. Figure 6.13 illustrates the method of hybridoma production. B cells, induced to divide and produce antibody by stimulation with a particular antigen, are fused with the cells of a plasmacytoma line (usually antibody non-secreting) adapted to continuous growth in culture. The resulting hybridoma cells possess properties of both partners in the fusion and thus can divide repeatedly but also secrete antibodies specific for the immunizing antigen. These hybridomas, like the original antigen-specific B cells, will be polyclonal, but individual clones can be isolated by culturing the cells singly and identifying the resulting monoclonal cell lines producing antibody of the desired specificity.

The usefulness of monoclonal antibodies derives from their clearly defined specificity, potentially limitless supply, and ease of production from established hybridomas. Examples of their uses include assays for the detection of microbes and the enumeration of cells expressing particular surface markers (e.g. the CD molecules of leucocytes, see p. 43). Monoclonal antibodies are also used clinically, e.g. administration of anti-CD3 antibody to kidney transplant patients to inhibit T cells causing acute rejection (see p. 269).

KEY POINTS

1 The typical immunoglobulin is composed of two identical heavy chains and two identical light chains. The amino-terminal variable domains of a heavy and a light chain form an antigen-combining site within one of the two Fab portions of the molecule. The Fc portion is composed of the heavy chain constant regions on the carboxy-terminal side of the hinge region.

2 The variable domains constitute the idiotype of an immunoglobulin, and form the antigen-combining site lined by hypervariable regions which are complementary to the specific epitope.

3 Affinity defines the strength of interaction between a single antigen-combining site and an epitope, whereas avidity refers to the cumulative interactions of several combining sites with an antigen.

4 Immunoglobulin isotypes (i.e. classes and subclasses) are defined by differences in their heavy chain constant regions. These determine their biological characteristics e.g. complement activation, cellular association via Fc receptors, and tissue distribution.

5 Immunoglobulin variable domains are encoded by numerous V, D and J exons whose diversity of selection, junctional variation, V_H/V_L combination and somatic mutation among different B cells generates

Continued

KEY POINTS

the enormous repertoire of antigen-combining sites. Similar mechanisms (with the exception of somatic mutation) generate the diversity of T cell receptors for antigens.

6 DNA rearrangements to bring the expressed heavy chain V–D–J exon combination into proximity with a different heavy chain constant region gene result in switching to the immunoglobulin class encoded by that gene.

7 The ability of antibodies to cross-link with antigens to form immune complexes is utilized in precipitation and agglutination assays. Other assays to detect antibody binding involve complement fixation or other measurable detection systems (e.g. involving fluorescent dyes, enzyme activities or radioisotopes).

8 The technology to produce monoclonal antibodies from B cell hybridomas has facilitated many studies in biology and medicine.

Further reading

Burton D.R. & Woof J.M. (1992) Human antibody effector function. *Advances in Immunology*, **51**, 1–84.

Miletic V.D. & Frank M.M. (1995) Complement–immunoglobulin interactions. *Current Opinion in Immunology*, **7**, 41–47.

Natvig J.B. & Turner M.W. (1993) The immunoglobulins. In Lachmann P.J., Peters D.K., Rosen F.S. & Walport M.J. eds, *Clinical Aspects of Immunology*, 5th edn. Blackwell Scientific Publications, Oxford.

Shakib F. ed. (1990) *The Human IgG Subclasses. Molecular Analysis of Structure, Function and Regulation*. Pergamon Press, Oxford.

Van de Winkel J.G.J. & Capel P.J.A. (1993) Human IgG Fc receptor heterogeneity: molecular aspects and clinical implications. *Immunology Today*, **14**, 215–221.

CHAPTER 7

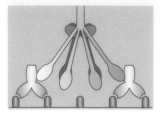

Complement

The presence of serum factors which could augment the effects of antigen–antibody combination was first detected by Jules Bordet almost 100 years ago. He showed that serum containing a red cell antibody would cause lysis of red cells when it was fresh but only agglutination when aged (Table 7.1). The material which *complemented* the effect of antibody could be restored by the addition of fresh non-antibody-containing serum and is now known to consist of a number of different plasma proteins which operate as an enzyme cascade similar to the coagulation system.

Most attention used to be focused upon the lytic ability of the complement system but this is now known to be one of several important biological effects of complement activation. Most of these involve the activation or fixation of the third complement component (C3) and this can be achieved in two different ways: by **activation** of the **classical pathway** or by **stabilization** of the **alternative pathway** (Fig. 7.1). If these initial steps take place on a cell or basement membrane then complement activation will proceed via the **membrane attack pathway** with the production of lytic lesions. Figure 7.2 gives an overview of the complement cascade.

The classical pathway (Fig. 7.3)

The first step involves the generation of an enzyme, C1 esterase, following a complex interaction between the three subunits of the first complement component C1 (C1q, C1r and C1s). The C1q molecule resembles a bunch of tulips and the critical requirement for C1 activation is that at least two of the six 'flower heads' of the C1q molecule interact with the $C_\lambda 2$ domain of two adjacent IgG molecules (Fig. 7.4) or two comparable complement-activating sites in the $C_\mu 3$ domain of two adjac-

EXPERIMENTS WITH RED CELLS

RBC	RBC antibody	C	Result
Present	Present	–	Agglutination
Present	Present	Present	Lysis
Present	–	Present	No effect

Table 7.1 Incubation of red cells with combinations of antibody and complement (C).

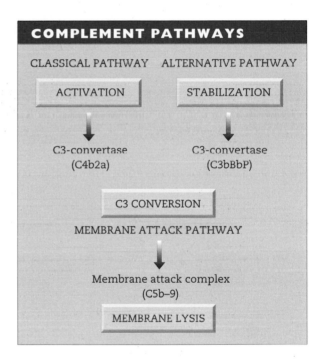

COMPLEMENT PATHWAYS

CLASSICAL PATHWAY   ALTERNATIVE PATHWAY

ACTIVATION   STABILIZATION

C3-convertase   C3-convertase
(C4b2a)   (C3bBbP)

C3 CONVERSION

MEMBRANE ATTACK PATHWAY

Membrane attack complex
(C5b–9)

MEMBRANE LYSIS

Fig. 7.1 Pathways of complement activation. See Fig. 7.2 and text for greater detail.

ent subunits of a single pentameric IgM molecule. In either case, these critical requirements are only fulfilled when the immunoglobulin is in complexed or aggregated form and this prevents the inappropriate activation of C1 by uncomplexed antibody.

The conformational change induced results in activation of C1r, which then activates C1s to form the esterase (C$\overline{1}$s). This enzyme acts on the next component in the sequence, C4, to yield a small fragment C4a and a larger fragment C4b. The latter binds covalently to membranes in the immediate vicinity but with a short half-life. C4b binds C2 in the presence of magnesium ions, causing the C2 molecule to become susceptible to the action of C$\overline{1}$s which cleaves it to form C2a and C2b. C2a remains

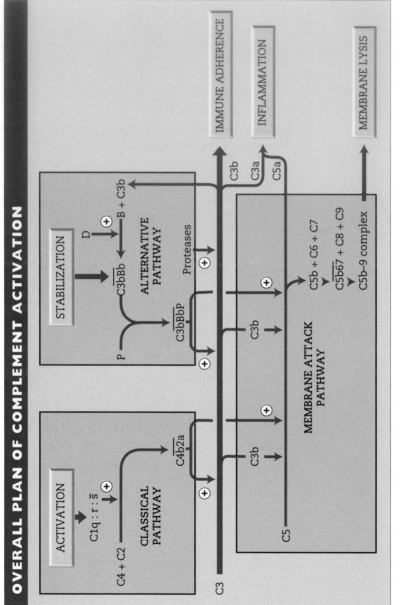

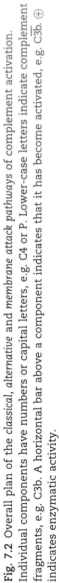

Fig. 7.2 Overall plan of the classical, alternative and membrane attack pathways of complement activation. Individual components have numbers or capital letters, e.g. C4 or P. Lower-case letters indicate complement fragments, e.g. C3b. A horizontal bar above a component indicates that it has become activated, e.g. C3b. ⊕ indicates enzymatic activity.

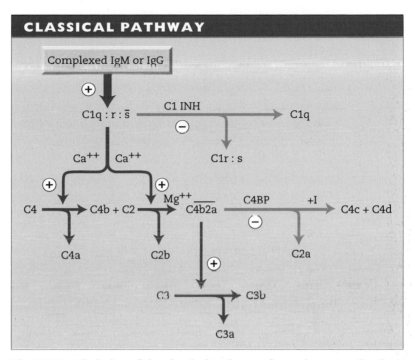

Fig. 7.3 Detailed plan of the classical pathway of complement activation. Ca++ and Mg++ indicate a requirement for divalent calcium and magnesium ions. See Table 7.2 for the full names of inhibitors. ⊕ indicates enzymatic activity; ○ indicates the action of inhibitory proteins.

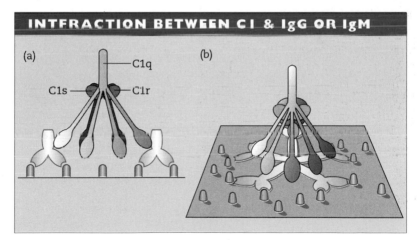

Fig. 7.4 Interaction between C1 and antigen-bound antibodies.
(a) Binding of C1q to the $C_\lambda 2$ domains of two adjacent IgG molecules.
(b) Binding of C1q to the $C_\mu 3$ domains of a pentameric IgM molecule.

attached to C4b on the surface membrane and this complex, designated $\overline{\text{C4b2a}}$, functions as a **C3 convertase** with a half-life of about 5 minutes at 37°C (Fig. 7.3).

The classical pathway can be activated by factors other than immunoglobulins, e.g. mannan-binding protein (whose three-dimensional structure is similar to that of C1q), C-reactive protein, lipid A of bacterial endotoxins, polyanions, polycations and some virus membranes.

Strict control of complement activation is necessary to limit complement-mediated tissue damage. Classical pathway activation is regulated by several inhibitors (Table 7.2), e.g. **C1 esterase inhibitor** (C1INH), which inactivates $\overline{\text{C1r}}$ and $\overline{\text{C1s}}$ as well as other serine esterases present in plasma. The combined activities of a **C4-binding protein** (C4BP) and **factor I** limit the effect of $\overline{\text{C4b2a}}$. C4BP accelerates the dissociation of $\overline{\text{C4b2a}}$ and facilitates the cleavage of C4b by I (Fig. 7.3 & Table 7.2).

C3 CONVERSION

This is the bulk reaction of the complement pathway during which several biological activities are generated. **C3 convertases** ($\overline{\text{C4b2a}}$ or $\overline{\text{C3bBbP}}$ described below) cleave C3 to give a small C3a fragment and a larger C3b fragment. C3a stimulates inflammation by causing degranulation of basophils and mast cells and is chemotactic for neutrophil polymorphs (Table 7.3): for these reasons C3a (together with C5a and C4a, which

INHIBITORS OF COMPLEMENT ACTIVATION

Mechanism of inhibition	Mediator of inhibition
Dissociation of the C1q:r:s complex	C1 inhibitor (C1 INH)
Dissociation of $\overline{\text{C4b2a}}$	C4 binding protein (C4BP) also Complement receptor 1 (CR1) also Decay-accelerating factor (DAF)
Dissociation of $\overline{\text{C3bBb}}$	Factor H (H) also Complement receptor 1 (CR1) also Decay accelerating factor (DAF)
Breakdown of C4b and C3b	Factor I (I), with membrane cofactor protein (MCP), C4BP, H, and CR1
Inhibition of C9 assembly with C5b-8	CD59

Table 7.2 Inhibitors of complement activation.

have similar properties) is referred to as an **anaphylatoxin** (anaphylaxis being a term used to describe the acute effects of mast cell degranulation (described in Chapter 9)).

C3b has a transient ability to form covalent bonds with membrane surfaces where it can act in concert with either of the two C3 convertases ($\overline{C4b2a}$ or $\overline{C3bBbP}$) to trigger the membrane attack pathway by interacting with C5 (Fig. 7.2). C3b is inactivated by a combination of **factor I** and **factor H** which yields iC3b. This converts, after cleavage by trypsin-like enzymes, to C3d and C3c (Table 7.2).

C3b and iC3b also mediate the phenomenon of **immune adherence** by their ability to bind to **C3 receptors** on phagocytes (neutrophils and macrophages). In this way, the coating or **opsonization** of antigens by C3b facilitates their phagocytosis (see Chapter 8).

Solubilization of immune complexes

Immune complexes have a greater tendency to aggregate if formed under conditions of complement depletion. The presence of an intact classical pathway retards precipitation and, activation of the alternative pathway and the interposition of C3b into the antigen–antibody lattice is required for solubilization to persist. Complexes containing C3b bind to complement receptors on red blood cells which transport them to the liver and spleen where macrophages remove the complexes from the red cell surface. The complement system thus has an important role in the processing of immune complexes to enable them to be cleared by the mononuclear phagocyte system which promotes the generation of B cell

SEQUELS TO COMPLEMENT ACTIVATION		
Function	**Mediators**	**Mechanisms**
Inflammation	C5a > C3a > C4a	Stimulation of mediator release by mast cells Attraction of neutrophils Activation of neutrophils
Immune adherence	C3b, iC3b > C4b	Binding to complement receptors Stimulation of phagocytosis Clearance of immune complexes
Membrane damage	C5b-9	Insertion of the membrane attack complex into lipid membranes

Table 7.3 Biological sequels to complement activation.

memory following the uptake of complexes in germinal centres. This role of complement may also explain the link between genetically determined complement deficiencies and a predisposition to immune complex disease.

The alternative pathway (Fig. 7.5)

Another kind of C3 convertase can be formed by the stabilization of a different set of proteins (but which includes C3b itself—a product of the classical pathway). Even in the absence of classical pathway activation, a degree of C3 conversion occurs due to spontaneous hydrolysis and this is enhanced by other proteases, e.g. plasmin, or other inflammatory products. This low-level or **tick-over** C3 conversion makes it possible for the alternative pathway to operate without activation of earlier components of the classical pathway. However, the complex which C3b forms with factor B in the presence of the protease factor D, i.e. C3bBb, rapidly dissociates unless factors are present which can stabilize

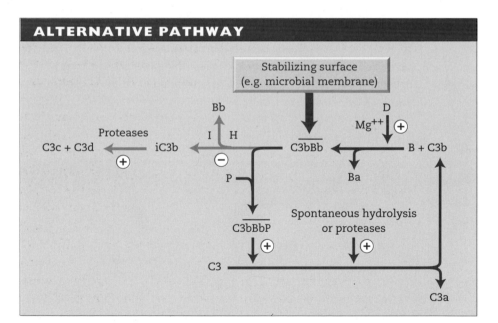

Fig. 7.5 Detailed plan of the alternative pathway of complement activation. Mg^{++} indicates a requirement for divalent magnesium ions. See Table 7.2 for the full names of inhibitors. ⊕ indicates an enzymatic activity; ⊖ indicates the action of inhibitory proteins.

it. These factors include microbial polysaccharides such as endotoxin, zymosan, sialic acid-deficient erythrocytes, nephritic factor, aggregrated forms of IgA and some subclasses of IgG (see Table 6.1).

The inhibitory factor H constantly acts to dissociate $\overline{\text{C3bBb}}$ (Table 7.2) but its affinity for C3b is considerably reduced when these stabilizing factors are present. They offer a protected surface which shields $\overline{\text{C3bBb}}$ from the inhibitor and permits its interaction with another alternative pathway protein – **properdin** (P) – to form the stable **alternative pathway convertase** $\overline{\text{C3bBbP}}$, which then acts on C3 (and C5) in equivalent fashion to $\overline{\text{C4b2a}}$. Indeed, C4 and C3 are structurally and functionally homologous, as are C2 and factor B. Thus, the alternative pathway takes the form of a feedback loop that operates whenever C3b is formed and is sustained when factors are present to stabilize the assembly of its C3 convertase.

The membrane attack pathway (Fig 7.2)

When C3b binds to surfaces in close proximity to either of the two C3 convertases described above, the membrane attack pathway is set in train following cleavage of C5. However, only the first step, in which C5 is cleaved to form C5a and C5b, is enzymatic.

C5a is the most potent of the anaphylatoxins and activates neutrophil polymorphs as well as mediating mast cell degranulation and neutrophil chemotaxis (Table 7.3). Both C3a and C5a are inactivated by a carboxypeptidase.

C5b has a labile binding site for cell membranes and binds C6 to form the stable complex C5b6 which then combines spontaneously with C7 to form $\overline{\text{C5b67}}$. $\overline{\text{C5b67}}$ has a short half-life but will bind to lipid membranes in the immediate vicinity. C8 binds to this complex, which inserts itself into cell membranes. Incorporation of C9 into the complex causes further penetration of the lipid bilayer and results in osmotic lysis of the cell. The fully developed lytic lesion – known as the **membrane attack complex** (MAC) – is a polymerized form of 10–16 C9 molecules and has the appearance of a plug or rivet in the electron microscope (Fig. 7.6). This mechanism of cell disruption shows interesting similarities with cell-mediated cytotoxicity (see Chapter 11). The promiscuous binding of C5b67 to cell membranes can result in tissue damage, known as **reactive lysis**. However, this is limited by a protein called **CD59** expressed on tissue cells which inhibits the association of C9 with C5b–8.

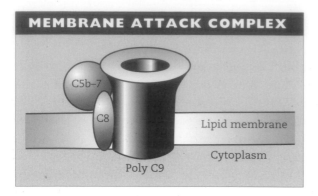

Fig. 7.6 The membrane attack complex of complement.

INADEQUATE REGULATION OF COMPLEMENT ACTIVATION

Hereditary angio-oedema

C1 esterase inhibitor acts on various serine esterases including $C\overline{1r}$, $C\overline{1s}$, plasmin and kallikrein. A deficiency of this enzyme is associated with acute attacks of angio-oedema which may follow minor trauma. C1 esterase inhibitor is important in controlling the action of plasmin and kallikrein in extravascular sites and in its absence the uncontrolled activation of C4 and C2 or of kininogen to bradykinin will occur with major effects on capillary permeability. This process does not cause effective C3 conversion as it mostly occurs in fluid phase without the generation of a stable membrane-bound C3 convertase.

Paroxysmal nocturnal haemoglobinuria

This disease occurs in patients with deficiencies in expression of decay-accelerating factor and CD59. The inadequate control of C3-convertase activity and MAC assembly results in intravascular red cell lysis.

Nephritic factor

This is an IgG molecule with specificity for $C\overline{3bBb}$ and is present in the sera of most patients with mesangiocapillary glomerulonephritis or partial lipodystrophy. Its presence is usually associated with marked depletion of C3, evidence of alternative pathway activation and normal levels of C1, C4 and C2. As the reactivity of this antibody resides in its Fab portion it is regarded as an autoantibody although purified nephritic factors have been shown to be larger than normal IgG and have an increased carbohydrate content. IgG antibodies reactive with the classical pathway C3 convertase $C\overline{4b2a}$ have been described in postinfective nephritis and systemic lupus although the link between infection and the development of these autoantibodies is unclear.

COMPLEMENT POLYMORPHISMS AND DEFICIENCIES

Heritable allotypic variation has been identified for many of the complement components (e.g. C4, C2, C3, C5, C6, C7, C8, factor B and factor D) and the loci for genes coding for C4, C2 and factor B are found in close association within the HLA complex (see Chapter 2). It is possible that some of the associations between certain HLA haplotypes and particular diseases may operate through functional differences in these variant complement proteins, particularly when there is little or no functional activity, e.g. as with the C4 null gene (see Chapter 16). Deficiencies of most of the individual complement components have been described and are briefly reviewed in Chapter 13.

KEY POINTS

1 Complement consists of a number of plasma proteins which operate as an enzyme cascade giving rise to various biological activities.
2 The complement system can be triggered via the classical pathway of C1 activation by antigen–antibody complexes leading to formation of the C3-convertase C4b2a, or via the alternative pathway involving stabilization of the C3-convertase C3bBbP on microbial surfaces.
3 The central event in complement activation is the conversion of C3 into C3a and C3b, which then activates the membrane attack pathway.
4 The biological activities resulting from complement activation are immune adherence (C3b binding to complement receptors), inflammation (C5a and C3a stimulating mast cells and neutrophils), and membrane lysis (by the membrane attack complex C5b–9).
5 Regulatory proteins limit inappropriate complement activation by causing dissociation or degradation of activated components. Inadequate regulation or inappropriate activation of complement can damage host tissues.

Further reading

Miletic V.D. & Frank M.M. (1995) Complement–immunoglobulin interactions. *Current Opinion in Immunology*, **7**, 41–47.

Morgan B.P. (1990) *Complement. Clinical Aspects and Relevance to Disease.* Academic Press, London.

Tomlinson S. (1993) Complement defense mechanisms. *Current Opinion in Immunology*, **5**, 83–89.

Walport M.J. & Lachmann P.J. (1993) Complement. In Lachmann P.J., Peters D.K., Rosen F.S.

& Walport M.J. eds, *Clinical Aspects of Immunology*, 5th edn. Blackwell Scientific Publications, Oxford.

Wetsel R.A. (1995) Structure, function and cellular expression of complement anaphylatoxin receptors. *Current Opinion in Immunology*, **7**, 48–53.

CHAPTER 8

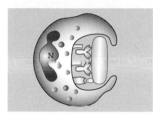

Phagocytes

Metchnikoff coined the terms 'macrophage' and 'microphage' for the two main varieties of phagocyte and believed that they had a more important role in protective immunity than Ehrlich's serum factors (i.e. immunoglobulins). However, in 1903 Almroth Wright demonstrated that the effector function of phagocytes is triggered by immunoglobulins – a similar state of affairs to that already described for the interaction between complement and immunoglobulin molecules. The clearance function of phagocytic cells — studied largely by the use of vital dyes — was emphasized in the definition of the 'reticuloendothelial' system but in recent years this misleading term has been replaced by a return to a Metchnikovian division into **mononuclear phagocytes** and **neutrophil polymorphs**. Mononuclear phagocytes are given different names in different tissues (Table 8.1) and are often referred to, collectively, as the **mononuclear phagocyte system**. They differ in size and morphology from neutrophils and, in addition to their role as phagocytes, are also able to present antigen to T cells (see Chapter 4). When activated, they secrete many proteins.

Macrophages

Macrophages are released from bone marrow as immature monocytes and mature in various tissue locations where they reside for weeks or years. They accumulate slowly at sites of infection, respond to a variety of stimuli (including cytokines) and have considerable potential for synthesis, secretion and regeneration. **Azurophilic lysosomal granules**, which are more evident in monocytes than in mature macrophages, contain lysozyme, myeloperoxidase and acid hydrolases (Fig. 8.1). Macrophages also possess a non-specific esterase and produce various neutral proteases, e.g. collagenase, elastase and plasminogen activator.

PRODUCTS OF THE MACROPHAGE

Contents of azurophilic lysosomal granules
  Myeloperoxidase
  Lysozyme
  Acid hydrolases
    e.g. β-glucuronidase, phosphatase

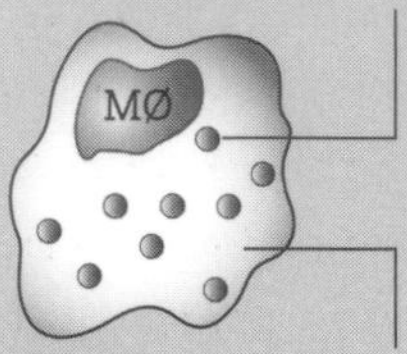

Other secreted products
  Complement components
    e.g. C1, C2, C3, C4, C5, B, D, properdin, I, H
  Neutral proteases
    e.g. collagenase, elastase, plasminogen activator
  Cytokines
    e.g. interleukins: IL-1, 6, 8, 10, 12
        tumour necrosis factor-α (TNF-α)
        colony stimulating factors (CSF)
        interferon-α (IFN-α)
  Fibronectin, α2 macroglobulin
  Coagulation factors
    e.g. tissue thromboplastin, V, VII, IX, X
  Prostaglandins
    e.g. PGE_2, $PGF_{2\alpha}$

Fig. 8.1 Stored and secreted products of the macrophage.

MONONUCLEAR PHAGOCYTES

Cell	Tissue
Monocyte	Blood
Macrophage	Bone marrow, spleen, lymph node medulla, lung (alveolar and pleural), peritoneum
Langerhans' cell	Skin
Veiled cell	Lymph
Interdigitating dendritic cell	Lymph node paracortex
Kupffer cell	Liver
Osteoclast	Bone
Type A cell	Synovium
Mesangial cell	Kidney
Microglial cell	Brain

Table 8.1 Cells of the mononuclear phagocyte system.

Other **secreted products** include many complement components (and inhibitors), coagulation factors, fibronectin, cytokines and prostaglandins, e.g. PGE_2 and $PGF_{2\alpha}$.

Neutrophils

Polymorphonuclear neutrophil leucocytes mature and are stored in bone marrow and are released rapidly into the circulation in response to various stimuli, notably bacterial infection. Neutrophils are 'end-cells' and only remain in the circulation for a few hours before they migrate into tissues where they die within 1–2 days. The functions of the neutrophil are mostly directed toward the killing and degradation of bacteria and are the major constituent of what, in the preantibiotic era, was known as 'laudable pus'. Their primary **azurophil lysosomal granules** contain several cationic proteins with antibacterial properties (the **defensins** and **serprocidins**) in addition to lysozyme, myeloperoxidase and acid hydrolases (Fig. 8.2). Unlike macrophages, they also possess **secondary specific granules** which contain lactoferrin (an iron-binding protein) as well as lysozyme, histaminase and transcobalamin II (a vitamin B_{12}-binding protein). Neutrophil polymorphs can also produce cytokines and are a potent source of leukotrienes, e.g. LTB_4—a chemotactic agent for polymorphs and monocytes—and LTC_4, LTD_4 and LTE_4 which together constitute **slow reacting substance** (SRS). They also produce prostaglandins, e.g. PGE_2, and platelet activating factor (PAF).

Common features of phagocyte responses

Both kinds of cell respond to infective stimuli with the following sequence of activities: chemotaxis, target recognition, ingestion, killing and degradation.

CHEMOTAXIS

Phagocytes exhibit directed movement along concentration gradients of chemotactic agents, e.g. **anaphylatoxins** (C3a, C5a), **leukotriene B4, interleukin-8** and phospholipids and peptides derived from bacteria. Neutrophils respond rapidly to these inflammatory stimuli by marginating to the walls of small blood vessels, adhering to endothelial cells and exiting into sites of inflammation (see Chapter 11).

PRODUCTS OF THE NEUTROPHIL

Contents of azurophilic granules
 Myeloperoxidase
 Lysozyme
 Acid hydrolases
  e.g. β-glucuronidase, phosphatase
 Cationic peptides (defensins)
  human neutrophil proteins - 1,2,3,4
 Cationic glycoproteins (serprocidins)
  elastase, cathepsin-G, proteinase-G, azurocidin

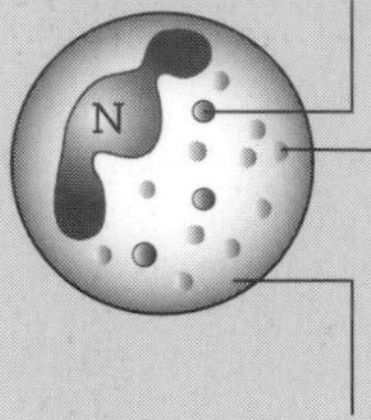

Contents of specific granules
 Lactoferrin
 Lysosyme
 Histaminase
 Transcobalamin

Other secreted products
 Cytokines
  e.g. interleukins: IL-1, 6, 8
    tumour necrosis factor-α (TNF-α)
    colony stimulating factors (CSF)
    interferon-α (IFN-α)
 Leukotrienes
  LTB_4
  LTC_4, LTD_4, LTE_4 (SRS)
 Prostaglandins
  e.g. PGE_2

Fig. 8.2 Stored and secreted products of the neutrophil.

TARGET RECOGNITION

Phagocytes can interact with targets hydrophobically or via specific sugar residues, e.g. mannose and glycan, or lipopolysaccharide for which they have receptors. However, target recognition is greatly enhanced when specific antibody of class IgG and/or C3b becomes fixed to the target surface, a process termed **opsonization** (Fig. 8.3). Both neutrophils and macrophages possess **Fc receptors** specific for IgG1 and IgG3 (see Table 6.2). Human polymorphs have 20 times as many receptors as macrophages and these receptors are more scarce on the immature monocyte. Neutrophil polymorphs also possess receptors of lower affinity for the Fc of IgA (Table 8.2). Both cells have receptors for C3b (**CR1**) and C3bi (**CR3** and **CR4**) which mediate the **immune adherence** phenomenon. CR3 and CR4 are members of the family of leuco-

Fc RECEPTORS ON EFFECTOR CELLS

	IgG1	IgG2	IgG3	IgG4	IgA1	IgA2	IgE
Macrophages	++	−	++	−	−	−	+
Neutrophils	++	+	++	+	+	+	−
Eosinophils	+	+	+	+	−	−	+

Table 8.2 Fc receptors on macrophages, neutrophils and eosinophils.

MICROBIAL PHAGOCYTOSIS & KILLING

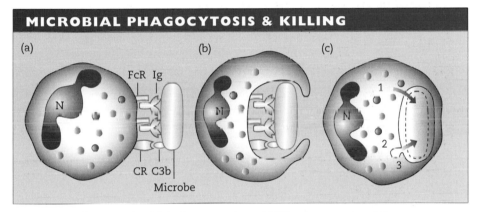

Fig. 8.3 Microbial phagocytosis and killing by a neutrophil.
(a) Recognition of a target opsonized by IgG antibodies and complement;
(b) ingestion of the target resulting in phagosome formation;
(c) degradation of the target in the phagolysosome: 1, neutral pH – toxic
oxygen compound; 2, alkaline pH – cationic proteins; 3, acidic
pH – lysosomal enzymes.

cyte integrins (see Chapter 11). The effective binding of complexed IgG
to Fc receptors on phagocytic cells is due to a cooperative effect between adjacent IgG molecules brought together in an immune complex
or other aggregated form as well as a conformational change in the
immunoglobulin Fc region with the expression of a new binding site. The
C3 receptor, on the other hand, only reacts with the converted C3b or
C3bi fragments. C3 receptors are particularly effective in promoting the
attachment of phagocytes to targets whereas Fc receptor binding induces
both phagocytosis and the respiratory burst which generates toxic oxygen compounds.

INGESTION

Phagocytosis is a form of localized endocytosis and contrasts with the
exocytotic process by which mast cells degranulate. It is an energy-

dependent process in which the plasma membrane gradually envelops the ingested particle and buds off the surface membrane internally to form a phagosome (Fig. 8.3). This then fuses with lysosomal granules to form the **phagolysosome** in which many of the processes take place which kill and degrade the ingested material (Fig. 8.3).

KILLING AND DEGRADATION
Oxygen-dependent mechanisms

Phagocytes contain both oxygen-dependent and oxygen-independent mechanisms for microbial attack (Table 8.3). Phagocytosis is accompanied by a burst of respiratory activity initiated by a membrane oxidase which reduces molecular oxygen to the **superoxide** anion (O_2^-) (Fig. 8.4). Most of the respiratory activity takes place within the hexose monophosphate shunt which provides NADPH as a fuel for the reduction of molecular oxygen. This process, which is initiated at the cell surface, continues on the inner surface of the phagolysosome. Superoxide is converted to **hydrogen peroxide** (H_2O_2) by spontaneous dismutation (predominantly at the cell surface) with the production of **singlet oxygen** ($^1O_2$) or by the action of superoxide dismutase (SOD) (present intracellularly) giving rise to molecular oxygen. Singlet oxygen is a highly reactive and unstable molecular species which emits light as it returns to ground state. This process can be measured by the technique of chemiluminescence. Hydrogen peroxide and superoxide also interact to form another extremely reactive species — the **hydroxyl radical** ($\cdot OH$). A major source of microbicidal activity develops in the phagolysosome when hydrogen

LYTIC MECHANISMS

Oxygen-dependent
Hydrogen peroxide
Singlet oxygen
Hydroxyl radical
Hypohalite
Nitric oxide

Oxygen-independent
Lysozyme
Lysosomal products
   cationic proteins (defensins, serprocidins)
   acid hydrolases
Lactoferrin (bacteriostatic)
Neutral proteases

Table 8.3 Lytic mechanisms of the phagocyte.

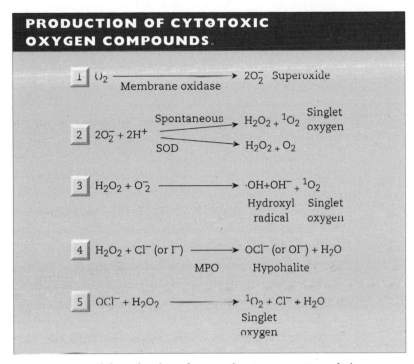

PRODUCTION OF CYTOTOXIC OXYGEN COMPOUNDS

1. $O_2 \xrightarrow[\text{Membrane oxidase}]{} 2O_2^-$ Superoxide

2. $2O_2^- + 2H^+ \overset{\text{Spontaneous}}{\underset{\text{SOD}}{\rightleftharpoons}}$
   $H_2O_2 + {}^1O_2$ Singlet oxygen
   $H_2O_2 + O_2$

3. $H_2O_2 + O_2^- \longrightarrow \cdot OH + OH^- + {}^1O_2$
   Hydroxyl radical   Singlet oxygen

4. $H_2O_2 + Cl^- \text{ (or } I^-) \xrightarrow[\text{MPO}]{} OCl^- \text{ (or } OI^-) + H_2O$
   Hypohalite

5. $OCl^- + H_2O_2 \longrightarrow {}^1O_2 + Cl^- + H_2O$
   Singlet oxygen

Fig. 8.4 Sequential production of cytotoxic oxygen compounds in phagocytic cells. SOD, superoxide dismutase; MPO, myeloperoxidase.

peroxide interacts with halide (Cl^- in the neutrophil and I^- in the macrophage) in the presence of **myeloperoxidase** (MPO) to form **hypohalite** and water. Hypohalite can then further react with hydrogen peroxide to form more singlet oxygen.

A variety of toxic materials are produced, therefore, during the oxidative burst. Several processes limit the spread of these toxic effects. **Catalase**, largely present in peroxisomes, converts hydrogen peroxide to water and oxygen; **superoxide dismutase** converts singlet oxygen to hydrogen peroxide, and hydrogen peroxide is also broken down by the glutathione redox system involving glutathione peroxidase. The chief extracellular antioxidant is caeruloplasmin, which has an equivalent role to that of superoxide dismutase within the cell. Caeruloplasmin is one of several acute phase proteins whose synthesis is considerably increased by the liver following the release of interleukin-1 (and see pp. 158–9).

Nitric oxide is another cytotoxic compound for which oxygen is a substrate. It is generated by neutrophils and some tissue cells via the action of nitric oxide synthetase (NOS) and the cofactor tetrahydrobiopterin (THBT) on L-arginine and O_2.

Oxygen-independent mechanisms

Ingested microbes become exposed to the contents of lysosomal granules when these fuse with the phagocytic vesicle. In the neutral to alkaline conditions of the newly formed phagolysosome, the most active components are the families of **basic cationic proteins** which act against both Gram-positive and Gram-negative organisms. The **defensins** (human neutrophil proteins-1, -2, -3 and -4) are cyclic peptides of 29–43 amino acids which insert into the membranes of their targets. The **serprocidins** are elastase, cathepsin G, proteinase G and azurocidin. Some, but not all of them, are serine esterases and their antibacterial properties are not dependent upon their enzymatic activity.

The pH drops within 10–15 minutes of phagosome–lysosome fusion. This acidic environment is itself detrimental to many microorganisms, and lysosomal enzymes become active: **lysozyme** hydrolyses the peptidoglycan of Gram-positive cell walls and **acid hydrolases** digest many constituents. **Lactoferrin** has a bacteriostatic effect due to its ability to bind iron strongly, thus making it unavailable to bacteria.

The killing activity of phagocytes is enhanced in the presence of certain cytokines. Interferon-γ (IFN-γ), a product of activated T cells and large granular lymphocytes, is particularly active and tumour necrosis factor-α (TNF-α) can act in conjunction with IFN-γ. TNF-α is produced by activated T cells, but also by macrophages when stimulated by certain bacterial products, e.g. lipopolysaccharide.

DEFICIENCY DISORDERS

The identity of the membrane oxidase which initiates the respiratory burst in phagocytic cells has been characterized as an NADPH oxidase and an associated flavin–cytochrome b complex. Patients with **chronic granulomatous disease** (CGD) lack this important enzyme and although their cells can phagocytose normally they are unable to kill most catalase-positive microorganisms, e.g. *Staphylococcus aureus* and *Serratia marcescens*. Catalase-negative organisms, e.g. streptococci, pneumococci and *H. influenzae*, are killed inside CGD phagocytes as they produce their own hydrogen peroxide which, as it is not broken down by microorganism-derived catalase, is able to join forces with the phagocyte's myeloperoxidase to generate hypohalite and a cidal effect.

C3 receptor deficiency has been described in individuals whose phagocytes can mount a normal respiratory burst and show normal IgG-dependent phagocytosis (e.g. of *Staph. aureus*) but impaired complement-dependent phagocytosis (e.g. of opsonized yeast). The C3bi (CR3) receptor is deficient whereas the C3b receptor (CR1) is normal, indicating the importance of the former in promoting this form of phagocytosis. Both these deficiencies are discussed further in Chapter 13.

KEY POINTS

1 Macrophages and neutrophils are called phagocytes because of their ability to ingest and destroy microbes.
2 Phagocytes produce a range of antimicrobial and inflammatory mediators. Some are stored in vesicles, e.g. azurophilic granules in both macrophages and neutrophils, and specific granules in neutrophils. Others are secreted.
3 Phagocytes migrate to sites of infection and inflammation in response to chemotactic signals.
4 Efficient target recognition by phagocytes involves binding to opsonized particles via Fc receptors and complement receptors.
5 Ingestion of microbes and formation of phagolysosomes activates oxygen-dependent and oxygen-independent mechanisms of killing.
6 Defects of the respiratory burst or complement receptor expression by phagocytes cause increased susceptibility to infection.

Further reading

Brown E.J. (1991) Complement receptors and phagocytosis. *Current Opinion in Immunology*, 3, 76–82.

Hellewell P.G. & Henson P.M. (1993) Neutrophils and their mediators. In Lachmann P.J., Peters D.K., Rosen F.S. & Walport M.J. eds, *Clinical Aspects of Immunology*, 5th edn. Blackwell Scientific Publications, Oxford.

Johnston R.B. (1993) Monocytes and macrophages. In Lachmann P.J., Peters D.K., Rosen F.S. & Walport M.J. eds, *Clinical Aspects of Immunology*, 5th edn. Blackwell Scientific Publications, Oxford.

Lewis C.E. & McGee J. O'D. eds. (1992) *The Macrophage*. IRL Press, Oxford.

Liew F.Y. & Cox F.E.G. (1991) Nonspecific defence mechanisms: the role of nitric oxide. *Immunology Today*, 12, A17–A27.

Nathan C.F. & Hibbs J.B. (1991) Role of nitric oxide synthesis in macrophage antimicrobial activity. *Current Opinion in Immunology*, 3, 65–70.

CHAPTER 9

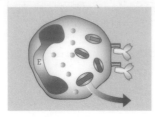

Mast Cells, Basophils and Eosinophils

Three kinds of granulocyte: mast cells, basophils and eosinophils, are distinguished from neutrophils by the differential staining characteristics of their granules. In mast cells and basophils this is due to the presence of an acidic proteoglycan; in eosinophils the characteristic granules contain several basic proteins. The basophil is a circulating cell whereas the mast cell is sessile and present throughout the body but chiefly in perivascular connective tissue, epithelia and lymph nodes. There is heterogeneity within the mast cell population and dye binding is considerably affected by the method of fixation as well as the individual stains used. In appropriately fixed sections, the granules of mucosal and connective tissue mast cells differ in their staining properties. Mucosal mast cells have some features in common with basophils (which contrast with connective tissue mast cells), i.e. they are smaller, short-lived, have chondroitin sulphate as acidic proteoglycan, are resistant to the inhibitory effect of sodium cromoglycate and require T cells for their growth and differentiation. Basophils have been identified in some forms of T cell-mediated immune responses, e.g. Jones–Mote or cutaneous basophil hypersensitivity (see Chapter 15), and the vagaries of fixation and staining techniques have probably caused them to be overlooked in other situations.

Mast cell **degranulation** has a general role in immunity by regulating the egress of inflammatory cells and molecules through endothelial tight junctions whenever a local inflammatory response is required to deal with a focus of infection (see Fig. 1.8 & Table 9.1). This increase in capillary permeability may be partly due to the contraction of endothelial cells similar to the effect on smooth muscle fibres elsewhere. It is likely that the remarkable variation in permeability that occurs in the postcapillary venule of the lymph node is regulated by a similar process of IgE or complement-mediated mast cell degranulation as mast cells are

EFFECTS OF MAST CELL MEDIATORS
Vasodilatation
Vascular permeability
Smooth muscle contraction
Leucocyte chemotaxis

Table 9.1 Inflammatory effects of mediators released by mast cells.

found plentifully at the cortico-medullary junction of lymph nodes, when appropriate fixation and staining methods are used. By contrast, the inappropriate activation of mast cells is one of the principal causes of allergic inflammation (see Chapters 14 and 15).

Triggering of mast cells and basophils

Mast cells and basophils possess surface **Fc receptors** with a high affinity for IgE ($Fc_\varepsilon RI$). Mast cells become activated either when surface-bound IgE molecules become cross-linked by antigen (or experimentally by anti-IgE) or following the local release of the **anaphylatoxins** C3a or C5a for which mast cells also bear receptors. In either case, a complex series of events follows in which various membrane enzymes are activated, calcium ions enter the cell, and granules and their preformed mediator contents are released by exocytosis (Fig. 9.1). New mediators generated from arachidonic acid metabolism are released over a longer time-scale, and were traditionally referred to as **slow reacting substance** of anaphylaxis (SRS).

The initial step involves the activation of a serine esterase followed by the activation of methyl transferases acting on membrane phospholipids, on the one hand, and adenyl cyclase which generates an increase in intracellular cyclic AMP and protein kinase activity, on the other. Phospholipid methylation and the action of phospholipases also lead to protein kinase activation (through the generation of diacyl glycerol) and are associated with three other important events: the opening of membrane **calcium channels** and the release of **intracellular calcium** (the latter occurring via the generation of inositol triphosphate); the generation of **fusagenic lipids** which encourage the fusion of perigranular and cell surface membranes, and the production of a supply of **arachidonic acid** from which various newly synthesized mediators are derived. The

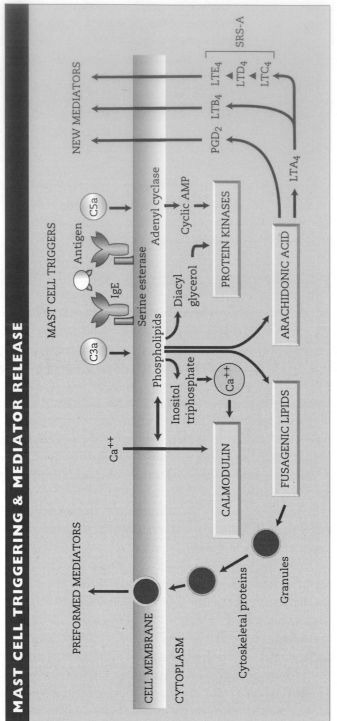

Fig. 9.1 Processes involved in mast cell triggering and mediator release. See text for further details.

activation of adenyl cyclase is critical for mediator release although its inhibition does not prevent phospholipid methylation. Once calcium enters the cell it is bound by calmodulin, which increases the activity of various enzymes (including protein kinases) and promotes the processes by which cytoskeletal proteins cause the contraction of microfilaments, leading to the extrusion of the granules and their contents. The anti-allergic drug **sodium cromoglycate** blocks mast cell degranulation and is thought to act by preventing the transmembrane influx of calcium ions.

Mast cell mediators (Fig. 9.2)

PREFORMED MEDIATORS

The preformed mediators present within mast cell granules consist of **histamine**, eosinophil and neutrophil **chemotactic factors** (ECF and NCF), a proteoglycan, acid hydrolases (e.g. aryl sulphatase and β-glucuronidase) and neutral proteases (e.g. tryptase and chymase) (Fig. 9.2). Histamine is a small molecule which contracts smooth muscle and

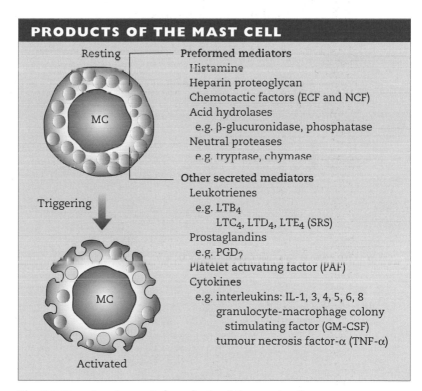

Fig. 9.2 Stored and secreted products of the mast cell.

increases vascular permeability. It is present in mast cell granules as part of a protein complex containing the proteoglycan **heparin**. Heparin is replaced by **chondroitin sulphate** in the basophil. Heparin is anticoagulant and anticomplementary and may have a role in promoting the diffusion of mast cell mediators following degranulation despite activation of the coagulation pathway, as well as contributing to the packaging and stabilization of mediators within the granules. The chemotactic factors released by mast cells not only attract other granulocytes but also increase the expression of their C3 receptors and have a stimulatory effect on the respiratory burst and the generation of oxygen-derived products.

SECONDARY MEDIATORS

SRS release takes place at a slower tempo than histamine release, the latter being a preformed mediator whereas the former has to be freshly synthesized. These 'secondary' mediators are lipid derivatives of **arachidonic acid** formed via two different pathways of metabolism under the control of cyclo-oxygenase and lipoxygenase enzymes (Figs 9.3 & 9.4). They include **SRS** (now known to consist of a combination of three different **leukotrienes**: LTC_4, LTD_4 and LTE_4); LTB_4 — a potent chemotactic agent; the prostaglandins PGE_2, PGD_2 and $PGF_{2\alpha}$, and platelet activating factor (PAF). The microsomal enzyme **cyclo-oxygenase**

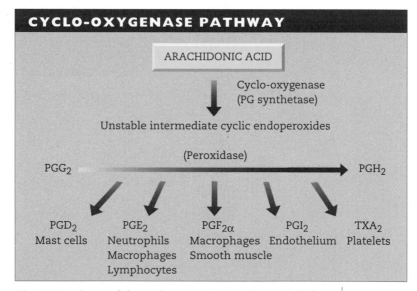

Fig. 9.3 Products of the cyclo-oxygenase pathway and the cell types in which they are formed.

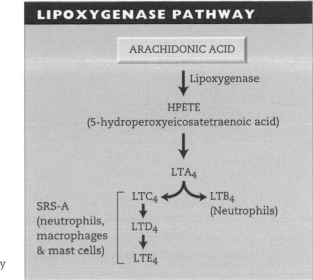

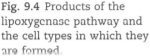

Fig. 9.4 Products of the lipoxygenase pathway and the cell types in which they are formed.

(also called prostaglandin synthetase) converts arachidonic acid to unstable intermediate cyclic endoperoxides (PGG_2 and PGH_2) which are then further metabolized to form stable prostaglandin mediators specific for each cell type. The predominant prostaglandin formed in mast cells is PGD_2 which causes vasodilatation, contracts smooth muscle and is chemotactic for neutrophils. PGE_2 is produced in neutrophils, macrophages and lymphocytes and is a potent vasodilator. Macrophages also synthesize $PGF_{2\alpha}$ which contracts smooth muscle. Other stable prostaglandins produced by this pathway include thromboxane (TXA_2), formed in platelets, and prostacyclin (PGI_2), which is produced by endothelial cells.

The leukotrienes are derived from the metabolic oxidation of arachidonic acid by the **lipoxygenase** pathway in which the unstable 5-hydroperoxyeicosatetraenoic acid (HPETE) is converted initially to the leukotriene LTA_4, which, depending on the cell concerned, either metabolizes to LTB_4 (e.g. in neutrophils) or is converted by the SRS pathway to LTC_4, LTD_4 and LTE_4. This latter process occurs in various granulocytes and mononuclear cells and it is possible that at least two cell types are required for the full expression of leukotriene synthesis. SRS is a particularly potent constrictor of smooth muscle and a vasodilator; it also causes mucus secretion. PGD_2 is the major arachidonic acid metabolite formed in connective tissue mast cells whereas LTC_4 production is prominent in mucosal mast cells and basophils.

Platelet activating factors (PAF) are phospholipids which cause calcium-dependent release of histamine and 5-hydroxytryptamine (5HT) from platelets and are also able to degranulate neutrophils and contract smooth muscle. Platelets themselves may have more of an immunological role than previously thought. They have Fc receptors for both IgG and IgE. Activation via the IgG receptor causes release of 5HT whereas triggering by IgE generates oxygen metabolites which have a lytic effect on some parasites, e.g. schistosomes.

CYTOKINES

Activated mast cells secrete a number of proinflammatory cytokines, including tumour necrosis factor-α and chemokines (e.g. interleukin (IL)-8). They also produce IL-4, which promotes the switching of B cells to IgE production as well as Th2 cell development, and IL-5 which promotes the differentiation and activation of eosinophils.

Eosinophils

Eosinophils are distinguished by the striking affinity of their granules for acid or aniline dyes. They form a small proportion of peripheral blood leucocytes (1–5 per cent) but are more prevalent in tissues. They probably share a common precursor with the basophil and show a later differentiation stage in the blood comparable to macrophage activation. They become more plentiful (in blood and relevant tissues) in allergic and parasitic diseases and their functions can be divided into effects on parasites and the inflammatory process.

Various factors have been identified which promote eosinophil proliferation and differentiation, e.g. granulocyte–macrophage colony stimulating factor, interleukins 3 and 5 and other eosinopoietic factors. Eosinophils also show a brisk chemotactic response to several materials liberated during the immune response, e.g. **ECF** (from mast cells), C5a and certain chemokines. ECF and C5a display synergism in their chemotactic effects on eosinophils.

Eosinophils phagocytose poorly but degranulate promptly in the presence of chemotactic factors and when membrane-bound IgG or IgE is cross-linked by antigen, i.e. exocytosis is more marked than endocytosis following triggering of their surface membrane, in contrast to the neutrophil. Eosinophils have Fc receptors for both IgG and IgE isotypes (see Table 8.2), although the latter ($Fc_\varepsilon RII$) are of lower affinity than the IgE receptors on mast cells ($Fc_\varepsilon RI$), and, like neutrophils, they also possess C3b receptors. They are able to form phagolysosomes following membrane triggering but this phenomenon is much less marked than in the neutrophil, and eosinophils display only limited proteolytic activity. A prominent role of neutrophils is the intracellular digestion of microbes (e.g. bacteria) which are readily phagocytosed. Eosinophils are more effective in the extracellular digestion of infectious agents that are too large to be engulfed (e.g. parasitic worms like schistosomes and helminths) (Fig. 9.5). Some of the contrasting features of mast cells, eosinophils and neutrophils are summarized in Table 9.2.

EOSINOPHIL PRODUCTS (Fig. 9.6)

Eosinophils display an oxidative burst with generation of H_2O_2 and, probably, superoxide but it is uncertain whether they produce the other more lytic oxygen radicals found in the neutrophil (see Fig. 8.4). Eosinophil peroxidase (EPO) is different from myeloperoxidase (MPO)

MAST CELLS, EOSINOPHILS AND NEUTROPHILS

	Mast cells	Eosinophils	Neutrophils
Lifespan	Long-lived	Long-lived	Short-lived
Dynamics	Sessile	Mobile	Mobile
Chemotactic response		+++ (ECF, C5a, chemokines)	+++ (NCF, C5a, chemokines)
Degranulation response (exocytosis)	+++	+++	+
Phagocytosis (endocytosis)	–	+	+++
Lytic ability	–	+++ (basic proteins, O radicals)	+++ (lysosomal enzymes, O radicals)
Receptors for cell triggering	IgE C3a C5a	IgE IgG C3b	IgG IgA C3b
Biological role	Gatekeeper, pro-inflammatory	Antihelminth, pro- or anti-inflammatory	Antibacterial

Table 9.2 Contrasting features of connective tissue mast cells, eosinophils and neutrophils.

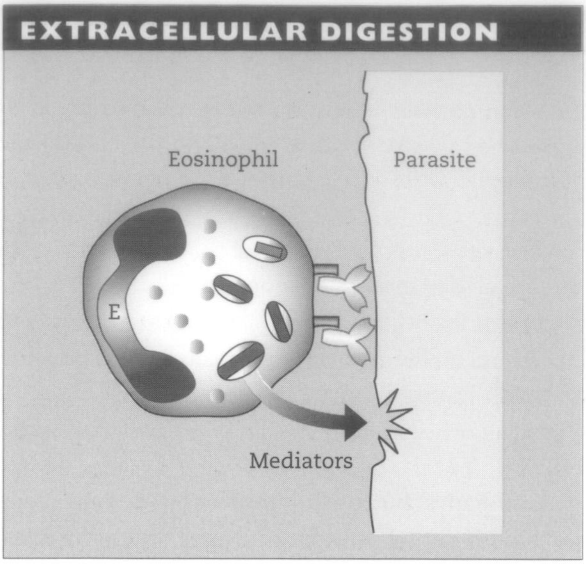

EXTRACELLULAR DIGESTION

Eosinophil

Parasite

E

Mediators

Fig. 9.5 Extracellular digestion by an eosinophil. The eosinophil is targeted to the surface of a parasitic worm opsonized by IgG or IgE antibodies. Lytic mediators are exocytosed on to the parasite surface (see text and Fig. 9.6).

PRODUCTS OF THE EOSINOPHIL

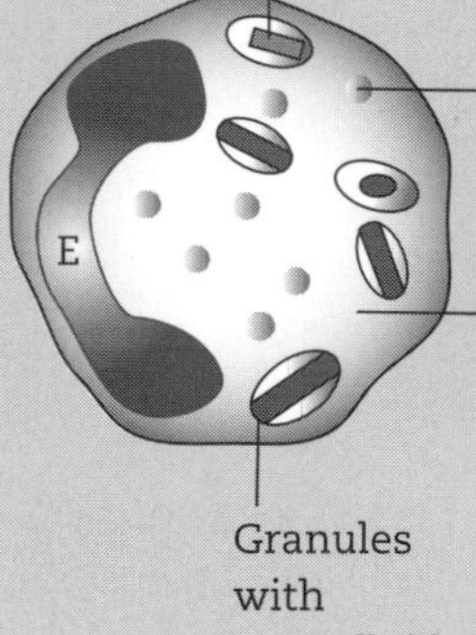

Contents of specific granules
Major basic protein
Eosinophil cationic protein
Eosinophil-derived neurotoxin
Eosinophil peroxidase

Contents of small granules
Aryl sulphatase
Acid phosphatase

Other mediators
Hydrogen peroxide, superoxide
Leukotrienes
 e.g. LTB_4, LTC_4
Prostaglandins
 e.g. PGE_2
Platelet activating factor
Cytokines
 e.g. interleukins: IL-1α, 3, 5, 6, 8
  granulocyte-macrophage colony
   stimulating factor (GM-CSF)
  tumour necrosis factor-α (TNF-α)
  transforming growth factors (α & β)
Enzymes
 e.g. histaminase
  phospholipase D
  β-glucuronidase

E

Granules
with
crystalloid
core

Fig. 9.6 Stored and secreted products of the eosinophil.

but may be able to work in concert with hydrogen peroxide and iodide or chloride ions to lyse some microorganisms, e.g. *Trichinella*. However, the major source of lytic activity in the eosinophil is the basic or **cationic proteins** contained within characteristic granules which are freely exocytosed during the degranulation response and are directly toxic to parasites, e.g. schistosomes, as well as to host cells.

The characteristic granules have a crystalloid core consisting largely of a **major basic protein** and a peripheral matrix containing other basic proteins, e.g. eosinophil cationic protein, and eosinophil-derived neurotoxin, as well as eosinophil peroxidase. Separate smaller granules contain aryl sulphatase and acid phosphatase. Eosinophil granules do not contain lysozyme. The exact location of other enzymes released by the cell, e.g. histaminase, β-glucuronidase and phospholipase D, is unclear. The protein which forms Charcot–Leyden crystals in various tissues and body fluids subjected to eosinophil degranulation is a lysophospholipase which resides in the plasma membrane of eosinophils (and basophils). Eosinophils also metabolize arachidonic acid to produce large amounts of platelet activating factor, leukotrienes, e.g. LTB_4 and LTC_4, and prostaglandin E_2. The cationic proteins and arachidonic acid metabolites derived from eosinophils contribute, together with mast cell products, to the acute and chronic phases of allergic inflammation. However, several of the other eosinophil products have an inhibitory effect on mast cell mediators (Table 9.3), and so may be anti-inflammatory.

Eosinophils also produce a number of cytokines (Fig. 9.6). Some of these act as autocrine growth factors (i.e. GM-CSF, IL-3 and IL-5), whereas others may have pro-inflammatory activity (e.g. IL-1, IL-6, IL-8, TNF-α) or anti-inflammatory effects (e.g. TGF-β).

MAST CELL:EOSINOPHIL INTERACTIONS

Inflammatory mediators produced by mast cells	Inhibitory factors produced by eosinophils
Histamine	Histaminase
	PGE_2
Heparin	Major basic protein
SRS	Aryl sulphatase
LTB	Peroxidase
PGD_2	
PAF	Phospholipase

Table 9.3 Interactions between mast cell and eosinophil products.

Hypereosinophilic syndrome

The release of inflammatory mediators can have serious complications in patients with the **hypereosinophilic syndrome** (HES). These consist of endomyocardial fibrosis and thromboembolic disease, largely associated with the liberation of toxic basic proteins and platelet activating factor, respectively.

KEY POINTS

1 Mast cells and basophils are activated by multivalent antigens cross-linking surface-bound IgE molecules, or by anaphylatoxins (C3a and C5a): this induces the release of inflammatory mediators.
2 Some mast cell mediators are preformed and stored in granules (e.g. histamine) and are exocytosed immediately upon activation. Other mediators are synthesized *de novo* (e.g. leukotrienes and prostaglandins). Mast cells also secrete cytokines.
3 Eosinophils possess granules containing lytic mediators (e.g. major basic protein) which are exocytosed upon interaction with IgE or IgG molecules bound to the surface of, for example, parasitic worms.
4 Eosinophils also secrete some mediators, which promote inflammation (e.g. arachidonic acid metabolites and cytokines) whereas others have anti-inflammatory effects on mast cell mediators.

Further reading

Holgate S.T. (1988) *Mast Cells, Mediators and Disease*. Kluwer Academic, London.

Schwartz L.B. (1993) Mast cells and basophils and their mediators. In Lachmann P.J., Peters D.K., Rosen F.S. & Walport M.J. eds, *Clinical Aspects of Immunology*, 5th edn. Blackwell Scientific Publications, Oxford.

Schwartz L.B. (1994) Mast cells: function and contents. *Current Opinion in Immunology*, **6**, 91–97.

Spry C.J.F. (1993) Eosinophils and their mediators. In Lachmann P.J., Peters D.K., Rosen F.S. & Walport M.J. eds, *Clinical Aspects of Immunology*, 5th edn. Blackwell Scientific Publications, Oxford.

Sutton B. & Gould H. (1993) The human IgE network. *Nature*, **366**, 421–428.

Weller P.F. (1994) Eosinophils: structure and functions. *Current Opinion in Immunology*. **6**, 85–90.

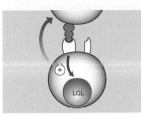

Killer Cells

Various cells of the immune system are able to inflict mortal damage on other living cells, e.g. bacteria, protozoa, the component cells of foreign grafts and even, in some circumstances, host tissues themselves. The ability of macrophages, neutrophils and eosinophils to release lytic oxygen radicals, lysosomal enzymes and toxic basic proteins has been reviewed in earlier chapters. Other cells, referred to here as **killer cells**, specialize in inflicting damage on **target cells** that represent a threat to the body, e.g. tissue cells which undergo malignant change or become infected. The latter applies particularly to viruses, but also to some intracellular bacteria (e.g. *Listeria monocytogenes*) and protozoa (e.g. *Toxoplasma gondii*). Killer lymphocytes may be of two types: **cytotoxic T (T_C) cells** and **large granular lymphocytes** (LGL). They differ in their mechanisms of target cell recognition but employ identical lytic mechanisms.

Mechanisms of target cell recognition

CYTOTOXIC T CELLS

T_C cells bear specific antigen receptors which bind to antigen associated with HLA molecules on the surface of target cells, as described in Chapter 4. Most T_C cells express CD8 and therefore interact with antigen bound to HLA class I molecules (Fig. 10.1a), but some CD4+ T cells can be cytotoxic for cells expressing HLA class II-associated antigens.

The differentiation of a cytotoxic precursor T cell (T_{CP}) into an active T_C cell requires help provided in the form of interleukin-2 (IL-2) released by a neighbouring T_H cell. It can also be achieved directly by interaction with a target cell if this expresses a sufficient quantity of adhesion molecules to stimulate the T_{CP} to make its own IL-2.

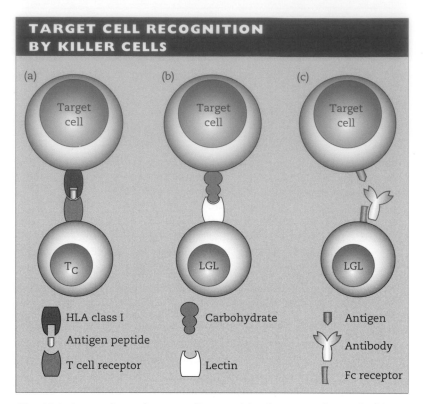

TARGET CELL RECOGNITION BY KILLER CELLS

(a)

Target cell

T_C

(b)

Target cell

LGL

(c)

Target cell

LGL

HLA class I

Antigen peptide

T cell receptor

Carbohydrate

Lectin

Antigen

Antibody

Fc receptor

Fig. 10.1 Comparison of target cell recognition by cytotoxic T cells (a), large granular lymphocytes mediating natural killer activity (b), and antibody-dependent cellular cytotoxicity (c). (a) The majority of T_C are CD8+ and recognize antigen associated with HLA class I. (b) The lectin: carbohydrate interaction involved in natural killer cell recognition is illustrated further in Fig. 10.2. (c) Antibody-dependent cellular cytotoxicity (ADCC) requires antibody to link the target to the killer cell by binding to antigen on the surface of the former and to the Fcγ receptor on the latter.

T_C cells have a key role in the lysis of host cells infected with budding viruses, i.e. those viruses which do not have a significant extracellular phase and are thus not amenable to the effects of antibodies working in conjunction with complement and phagocytes. The T cell killing of target cells involves three distinct phases:

1 Adhesion and recognition. A T_C cell initially binds to a potential target by adhesion molecules, i.e. CD2 and LFA-1 on the former binding to LFA-3 (lymphocyte function-associated antigen-3) and ICAM-1 (intercellular adhesion molecule-1), respectively, on the latter (see p. 55). If the target cell expresses antigen–HLA complexes which can engage specific antigen receptors on the cytotoxic T cell, then the cellular interaction becomes sufficiently strong and stable for killing to occur.

2 *Lethal hit.* The T_C cell contains cytotoxic mediators stored in cytoplasmic vesicles. These granules reorientate to the area of contact with the target cell and release their contents on to the target cell surface. Thus, although the cytotoxic mediators are not antigen-specific, they are directed against cells bearing the specific target antigens (e.g. viral components) so that innocent bystander cells are not damaged. Interactions between surface molecules of the T_C cell and the target cell also contribute to the death of the latter.

3 *Target cell death.* The mechanisms leading to the death of the target cell involve two complementary processes called **osmotic lysis** and **apoptosis**, which are described later in this chapter.

Once it has delivered the lethal hit, the T_C cell does not need to remain in contact with the target cell for death to ensue. Instead, the cytotoxic T cell can detach and **repeat** the process of killing against other cells expressing the target antigen.

LARGE GRANULAR LYMPHOCYTES

Natural killer cells are identified morphologically as **large granular lymphocytes** (LGL) by virtue of having more cytoplasm than resting T and B lymphocytes, and one or two large azurophilic granules (Table 10.1). Their presence and activity is readily detectable in peripheral blood and, to a lesser extent, in lymphoid organs. They are also called *natural killer cells* because they exhibit spontaneous killing against a variety of target cell types without the need for antigen-specific activation as required by T cells (Fig. 10.1b). However, their activity is greatly enhanced by exposure to certain cytokines, particularly type I interferons (IFN-α and β) produced by virus-infected cells, or by IL-12 secreted by activated macrophages and B cells. Activated LGL are themselves a potent source of IFN-γ.

LGL do not possess antigen-specific receptors, i.e. they do not rearrange genes encoding T cell receptors or immunoglobulins. The ways in which LGL recognize their targets are still being elucidated, but require that they distinguish their targets from normal cells. LGL possess carbohydrate-binding proteins on their surface, known as **lectins**, which can interact with certain carbohydrates normally expressed on cell surfaces (Fig. 10.2). This interaction alone would trigger the LGL to kill the cell to

CHARACTERISTICS OF LGL

Large azurophilic granules
Secondary lysosomes containing acid phosphatase
Absent peroxidase and non-specific esterase
Well-developed Golgi apparatus
Fc receptors for IgG1 and IgG3 (FcγRIII)
C3b receptors (CR3)
NK and ADCC activity
Non-T suppressor activity
Respond to IL-2, IL-12 and IFN-α/β
Produce cytokines: IFN-γ, TNF-α/β, IL-3, M-CSF, GM-CSF

Table 10.1 Characteristics of large granular lymphocytes.

which it binds. However, LGL also express other molecules which bind to HLA class I molecules on normal cells, and this interaction inhibits their cytotoxic activity (Fig. 10.2a). By contrast, this latter interaction may not occur with virus-infected cells, because their surface HLA class I molecules are altered or reduced in number, so the cell becomes a target of NK-mediated cytotoxicity triggered by the lectin–carbohydrate interaction (Fig. 10.2b).

Antibody-dependent cellular cytotoxicity

Antibody-dependent cellular cytotoxicity (ADCC) describes an alternative mechanism used by LGL to interact with their targets which involves the cooperation of antibodies. In addition to the adhesion molecules described above, LGL also express receptors for the Fc portion of IgG1 and IgG3 antibodies (Fc$_\gamma$RIII: see Table 6.2). Thus, antibodies bound to surface antigens of a target cell can facilitate the adhesion of LGL and the triggering of their cytotoxic activity (Fig. 10.1c). Although the relative importance of ADCC in immune defence is unclear, it may contribute to defence against enveloped viruses whose membrane proteins are expressed on the surface of infected cells during the process of budding.

Mechanisms of target cell killing

SECRETED PROTEINS

The cytoplasmic granules of both T$_C$ and LGL contain two types of cytotoxic proteins, called **perforins** and **granzymes**, which are rapidly secreted on to the surface of a target cell to which a killer cell binds. The

INTERACTIONS INVOLVED IN NK ACTIVITY

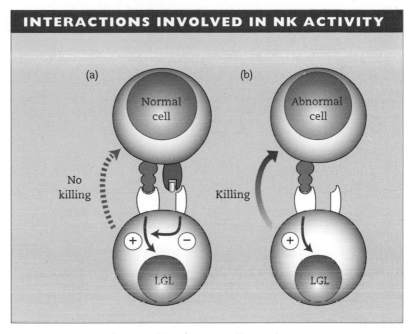

Fig. 10.2 Target cell recognition by LGL cells. Lectins on LGL bind to carbohydrates on other cells. LGL also express proteins which bind to HLA class I. The latter interaction inhibits the triggering of cytotoxic activity against normal cells (a), but not abnormal cells with reduced or altered HLA class I expression (b).

perforins are similar in structure and function to the complement proteins C6–C9 which form the membrane attack complex (see Chapter 7). In the presence of calcium ions, the perforin molecules polymerize to form tubular structures which insert into the lipid bilayer of the target cell, thus 'perforating' its membrane. This loss of membrane integrity may lead to the death of the target cell because of the disruption of normal ion gradients, or due to the passage of water into the cell through the perforin pores leading to **osmotic lysis** (Fig. 10.3).

Granzymes are serine proteases which exert their cytotoxic effects after entry into the target cell. Their entry is assisted by the perforins, possibly because granzymes pass through the perforin pores. Alternatively, the target cell may endocytose (i.e. engulf) areas of membrane damaged by perforins in an attempt to repair its surface. By so doing, it also takes up some of the extracellular fluid containing the granzymes. Once inside, granzymes induce the target cell death by activating the cell's own endonuclease enzymes which degrade its DNA. This mechanism of cell death is termed **apoptosis** (Fig. 10.3).

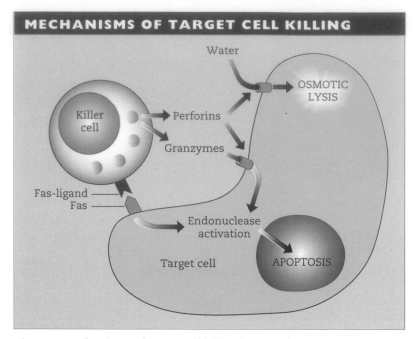

Fig. 10.3 Mechanisms of target cell killing by T_C and LGL.

MEMBRANE LIGANDS

In addition to the action of their granule components, killer cells are able to induce target cell death through the interaction of cell surface ligands. Many cells express a surface receptor protein called **fas**, and killer cells express a fas-binding protein. These two proteins are structurally related to the tumour necrosis factor (TNF) receptor and the TNF cytokine, respectively. When killer cells bind to their targets, the interaction of the fas ligand with fas induces apoptosis of the target cell.

Thus, killer cells have several weapons within their arsenal for ensuring the death of their target cells. They can 'execute' the target by damaging its surface membrane with perforins, or they can induce 'suicide' of the target through the effects of granzymes or by binding to fas.

Cooperation between killer cells and interferons

Effective defence against intracellular viruses requires contributions from both LGL and T_C cells in conjunction with interferons (IFN). Cytotoxic T cells are particularly efficient at killing virus-infected cells. However, the recruitment, activation and proliferation of T_C cells specific for antigens of the infecting virus may take several days, whereas LGL are spontane-

TYPE I AND TYPE II INTERFERONS

Interferon type	Cell source	Antiviral activity	Cells activated	Increased HLA expression
Type I (IFN-α/β)	Virus-infected cells	+++	LGL	Class I
Type II (IFN-γ)	Activated LGL and T cells	+	Macrophages	Class I and class II

Table 10.2 A comparison of type I and type II interferons.

ously active against infected target cells. LGL may act to limit virus spread during the early stages of infection until the T_C cells become fully activated and eliminate the virus. This is illustrated by a patient with NK cell deficiency, who suffered from repeated herpes virus infections which were severe initially but resolved after activation of the T cell response.

Cytokines are involved in killer cell functions, and the interferons are particularly important in antiviral immunity (Table 10.2). Type I interferons (IFN-α and IFN-β) are secreted by virus-infected cells and act from the early stages of a viral infection. Type II interferon (IFN-γ) is produced by activated LGL and T cells and contributes to the response once the killer cells become active. Both types of interferons have a direct antiviral effect by 'interfering' with the production of new virus particles. They do this by stimulating the cells to produce enzymes which degrade viral mRNA and inhibit protein synthesis.

Interferons also enhance LGL activity and target cell recognition by T_C cells (Table 10.2). Type I interferons directly activate LGL whereas IFN-γ stimulates macrophages which produce another LGL-activating cytokine, IL-12. Increased expression of HLA molecules is stimulated by interferons and enhances target cell presentation of viral antigens for recognition by T_C cells. Some viruses can suppress surface HLA expression by the cells they infect but this makes the cells better targets for killing by LGL.

KEY POINTS

1 There are two types of killer lymphocytes called cytotoxic T (T_C) cells and large granular lymphocytes (LGL). They are cytotoxic to target cells which have become infected or malignant.
2 Most T_C cells express CD8 and interact with target cells presenting specific antigens associated with HLA class I molecules.

Continued

KEY POINTS

3 LGL are large granular lymphocytes. They do not possess antigen-specific receptors but have surface lectins which interact with carbohydrates on target cells. The killing of normal cells is prevented by simultaneous interaction with HLA class I molecules.

4 LGL also have Fc-receptors which can interact with antibodies bound to target cell surface antigens, leading to antibody-dependent cellular cytotoxicity.

5 Both T_C and LGL possess granules containing cytotoxic proteins which are secreted on to the target cell surface. Perforins cause membrane damage and osmotic lysis whereas granzymes induce apoptosis of the target cell. Fas–fas ligand interaction between a target cell and killer cell can also cause target cell apoptosis.

6 The spontaneous cytotoxicity of LGL is important early on in intracellular viral infections, whereas viral clearance is dependent upon T_C cell activation. Interferons enhance killer cell functions as well as directly inhibiting viral replication.

Further reading

Lewis C.E. & McGee J.O'D. eds. (1992) *The Natural Killer Cell.* IRL Press, Oxford.

Liu C.-C., Walsh C.M. & Young J.D.-E. (1995) Perforin: structure and function. *Immunology Today*, **16**, 194–201.

Podack E.R. (1993) Killer and natural killer cells: functions of non-major histocompatibility complex-restricted killer cells. In Lachmann P.J., Peters D.K., Rosen F.S. & Walport M.J. eds, *Clinical Aspects of Immunology*, 5th edn. Blackwell Scientific Publications, Oxford.

Podack E.R. (1995) Execution and suicide: cytotoxic lymphocytes enforce Draconian laws through separate molecular pathways. *Current Opinion in Immunology*, **7**, 11–16.

Smyth M.J. & Trapani J.A. (1995) Granzymes: exogenous proteinases that induce target cell apoptosis. *Immunology Today*, **16**, 202–206.

Yokoyama W.M. (1995) Natural killer cell receptors. *Current Opinion in Immunology*, **7**, 110–120.

PART 2

Immunopathology

CHAPTER 11

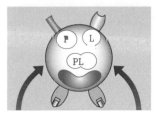

Immunity and Infection

Until recently, the view had become prevalent in developed countries that scourges of infection were a thing of the past. However, a quick look at the global pattern of morbidity, and the resurgence of various forms of infectious disease among the wealthier nations of the world, indicates that infection is still a major cause of disease. The balance between the adaptive immune response and the pathogenic onslaught it may face remains delicate in spite of the introduction of vaccines and many forms of antimicrobial chemotherapy. The complexity of the immune system is mirrored by the diversity of the pathogens that may interact with it. A schematic representation of host defence mechanisms, contained within their epithelial boundaries and surrounded by a universe of pathogens, is shown in Fig. 11.1. Each pathogen has its own life cycle, routes of transmission, and mechanisms for maintaining its survival within the hostile host environment.

Following the Second World War, and concern about infections such as poliomyelitis, influenza, malaria, smallpox and salmonellosis, various national centres were established to conduct surveillance of infectious (communicable) diseases, e.g. the Center for Disease Control in Atlanta and the Communicable Disease Surveillance Centre in London. A re-awakening of interest in, and concern about, infectious diseases has led more recently to the appointment of consultants in communicable disease control throughout the UK. The World Health Organization has coordinated measures toward the control and elimination of a number of important infectious diseases. Smallpox — already referred to in Chapter 1 — was eliminated in 1980 and plans are well advanced toward the

HOST DEFENCE MECHANISMS

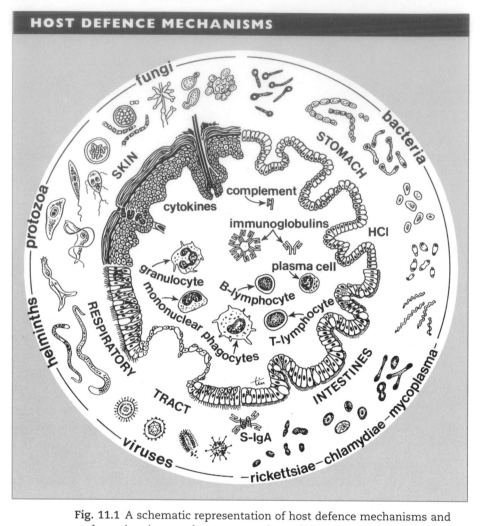

Fig. 11.1 A schematic representation of host defence mechanisms and pathogenic micro- and macro-organisms. (After Van Furth R. (1980) *Review of Infectious Diseases*, 2, 104–105 with permission.)

elimination of poliomyelitis by the year 2000. However, current global estimates suggest that 50 million people have tuberculosis, around 10 million are infected with malarial parasites, and more than 10 million individuals have contracted HIV infection since it was first recognized in 1981. New vaccines, chemotherapy, and effective public health measures are urgently required to combat these and other burdens of infectious disease.

A list of some important human pathogens and the diseases they cause is given in Table 11.1. However, the picture is not static and advances in microbiology, epidemiology and immunology have recently led to the

IMPORTANT HUMAN PATHOGENS

Organism	Disease
Bacteria	
Staphylococcus spp.*	Boils, septicaemia, food poisoning
Streptococcus spp.	Tonsillitis, erysipelas, scarlet fever, pneumonia
Bacillus anthracis	Anthrax
Corynebacterium diphtheriae	Diphtheria
Clostridium spp.	Tetanus, gas gangrene, botulism
Neisseria spp.	Meningitis, gonorrhoea
Escherichia coli	Urinary tract infection, gastroenteritis
Salmonella spp.	Enteric fever, food poisoning
Shigella spp.	Dysentery
Vibrio cholerae	Cholera
Proteus spp.	Urinary tract and wound infection
Haemophilus influenzae	Meningitis, pneumonia
Bordetella pertussis	Whooping cough
Yersinia pestis	Plague
Brucella spp.	Undulant fever
Mycobacterium spp.	Tuberculosis, leprosy
Legionella spp.	Legionnaires' disease
Treponema pallidum	Syphilis
Chlamydia spp.	Trachoma, pneumonia, genital tract infection
Viruses	
Polioviruses	Poliomyelitis
Hepatitis viruses (e.g. A, B, C)	Hepatitis
Rubivirus	Rubella
Measles virus	Measles
Mumps virus	Mumps
Respiratory syncytial virus	Bronchiolitis
Orthomyxoviruses	Influenza
Rhinoviruses, coronaviruses	Common cold
Rhabdovirus	Rabies
Papillomavirus	Warts
Herpes simplex virus	Herpes
Varicella-zoster virus	Chickenpox, shingles
Epstein–Barr virus	Infectious mononucleosis
Human immunodeficiency virus	AIDS
Flaviviruses	Yellow fever, dengue
Rotaviruses	Gastroenteritis
Fungi	
Candida albicans	Thrush, dermatitis
Dermatophytes (e.g. *Trychophyton* spp.)	Ringworm
Cryptococcus neoformans	Meningitis

Continued on p. 146

Table 11.1 Some important human pathogens.

IMPORTANT HUMAN PATHOGENS

Organism	Disease
Protozoa	
Plasmodia spp.	Malaria
Leishmania spp.	Leishmaniasis
Toxoplasma gondi	Toxoplasmosis
Trypanosoma spp.	Trypanosomiasis
Helminths	
Cestodes (e.g. *Taenia* and *Echinococcus* spp.)	Cysticercosis, hydatid disease
Trematodes (e.g. *Schistosoma* spp.)	Schistosomiasis (bilharzia)
Nematodes (e.g. *Ascaris, Necator, Wucheria, Onchocerca, Dracunculus* and *Toxocara* spp.)	Ascariasis, hookworm disease, filariasis, river blindness, guinea worm disease, toxocariasis (larva migrans)
* spp. indicates that multiple species cause disease.	

Table 11.1 (*continued*)

RECENTLY IDENTIFIED PATHOGENS

Organism	Disease
Borrelia burgdorferi	Lyme disease
Campylobacter jejuni	Enteritis
Escherichia coli 0157	Haemorrhagic colitis, haemolytic uraemic syndrome
Helicobacter pylori	Peptic ulceration, gastric cancer
Rochalimaea henselae	Cat scratch fever, bacillary angiomatosis
Cryptosporidium	Gastroenteritis
Hantaviruses	Haemorrhagic fever, renal and respiratory failure
Hepatitis D & E viruses	Hepatitis
Human herpes virus 6	Rash and fever
Parvovirus B19	Rash, arthropathy and aplastic anaemia
Small round structured viruses	Gastroenteritis

Table 11.2 Recently identified human pathogens.

identification of a number of 'new' pathogens, some of which are listed in Table 11.2.

Defence against infection

The requirements of an effective immune system are considerable and are dictated by the diversity of the pathogens that it may encounter (Table 11.3). These demands are met by multiple types of cells and molecules which respond dynamically and cooperate synergistically throughout the body. The activity of these components is carefully regulated to minimize damage to host tissues.

Thus, mammalian organisms have a powerful armoury of cells and molecules that can destroy most kinds of pathogen. These have been described in earlier chapters but are summarized diagrammatically in Fig. 11.2. They include complement activating proteins (e.g. C-reactive protein (CRP), mannose-binding protein (MBP), and antibodies of classes IgM, IgG and IgA); the alternative and classical complement pathways; phagocytic cells (e.g. polymorphonuclear leucocytes and macrophages); interferons and other cytokines, T and B lymphocytes, and natural killer cells.

The contribution of each component or set of components is optimized by having both **adaptive** and **innate** options for activation, which may generate **multiple effector functions** (Table 11.4). For

IMMUNOLOGICAL REQUIREMENTS

To recognize antigens contained within a vast repertoire of potential pathogens

To mount a large response to a small initial stimulus in order to overcome the rapid growth of many microbes

To destroy many very different types of pathogens

To minimize damage to host tissues

Table 11.3 Requirements of an effective immune system.

IMMUNOLOGICAL COMPONENTS

The component cells and molecules of the immune system are:
   multiple
   dynamic
   cooperative
   regulated

The components may be activated by innate or adaptive mechanisms

The activation of a component may generate multiple effects

Different components may have similar effects

Table 11.4 The nature of the components of an effective immune system.

MECHANISMS OF EVASION OF THE IMMUNE RESPONSE

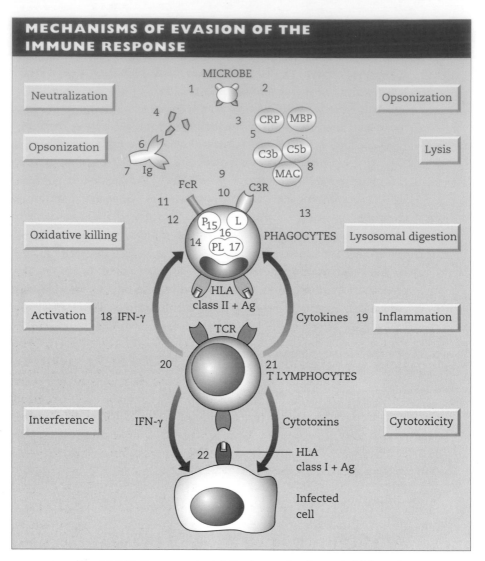

Fig. 11.2 Defences against infection and points at which pathogens may evade them (see p. 151–3 for description of mechanisms 1–22). CRP, C-reactive protein; MBP, mannan-binding protein; MAC, membrane attack complex; P, phagosome; L, lysosome; PL, phagolysosome).

example, the complement system may be activated by antigen–antibody complexes (via the classical pathway) or directly by microbial components (via the alternative pathway), generating inflammatory (C3a, C5a), opsonizing (C3b) and membrane damaging (C5b–9) activities.

Each process has its preferential targets, optima and kinetics but, in general, extracellular bacteria, viruses that have a viraemic phase (i.e.

spread through the blood stream), and some fungi, are susceptible to the effects of antibody, complement, and phagocytes whereas intracellular bacteria, some enveloped (or 'budding') viruses, protozoa and some other fungi can only be eliminated by the action of T cells, large granular lymphocytes (LGL) and macrophages. Macroparasite worms, i.e. helminths, are usually impervious to the effects of antibody and complement or lymphocyte-mediated cytotoxicity but are vulnerable to antibody-dependent reactions mediated by neutrophils, eosinophils and macrophages. These processes lead to recovery from a primary infection. Resistance to reinfection is usually mediated by IgG or IgA antibodies, though cell-mediated immunity is required to maintain resistance to some infections, e.g. tuberculosis.

Antibody molecules **neutralize** microbes in various ways: by inactivating microbial toxins, by preventing micro-organisms attaching to receptors on host cells, by inhibiting motility or by metabolic effects. The combination of immunoglobulin molecules with an invading microbe may also lead to uptake by phagocytes. This process of **opsonization** may follow the interaction of antigen: immunoglobulin complexes with Fc receptors on phagocytes, but it is considerably enhanced following complement activation and the interaction of C3b with C3 receptors on the phagocyte surface. The alternative and classical complement pathways may be activated by the surface components of microbes; by complexed antibody or other complement activating proteins (e.g. CRP, MBP), or by other means. This may cause **lysis** of the organism following the insertion of membrane attack complexes (MAC) formed from terminal components of the complement pathway (see Chapter 7).

Many pathogens that survive initial contact with this array of complement activating proteins are taken up into phagocytes and subjected to a process of **oxidative killing** within the phagosome. This is triggered by a membrane oxidase and results in the production of superoxide, singlet oxygen and hydroxyl radicals (see Chapter 8). The phagosome then fuses with lysosomal granules containing myeloperoxidase, lysozyme and acid hydrolases. Polymorph granules also contain neutral proteases and toxic cationic proteins. The presence of myeloperoxidase in the phagolysosome generates further microbicidal activity in the form of hypohalite.

The process of **lysosomal digestion** not only augments parasite killing but, in the macrophage, is a route for antigen presentation whereby antigenic epitopes are expressed on the cell surface in conjunction with HLA Class II glycoproteins and provide a signal for T cell stimulation. CD4$^+$ T cells then release interferon-γ which activates macrophages and has an inhibitory effect on many viruses and some other pathogens, e.g. mycobacteria and protozoa. Interferon induces the anti-viral state of **interference** by the action of two enzymes, a protein kinase and an oligoadenylate synthetase which inhibit the translation of viral RNA and protein synthesis. Interferon-γ also enhances HLA Class I and II expression on the surface of virus-infected cells and **activates** the phagocytic and digestive capacity of macrophages. Activated macrophages and stimulated T cells, LGL and B cells also produce a variety of other **cytokines** (e.g. interleukin-1 (IL-1), IL-2, IL-4, IL-6 and tumour necrosis factor (TNF)) which add to the intensity of the **inflammatory response** (see Chapters 4 & 5). Some intracellular pathogens are eliminated by the destruction of the cells they parasitize, and this **cytotoxicity** is mediated by cytotoxins secreted by NK cells and cytotoxic T cells.

This apparent superfluity of defensive mechanisms may seem inappropriate but recent work has demonstrated the extraordinary variety of mechanisms by which successful pathogens are able to evade the actions of the immune system. This helps to explain how the tempo and severity of an infection can vary from death within 24 hours (as in some cases of untreated meningococcal infection, streptococcal septicaemia or falciparum malaria), to slow but progressive infection with *Mycobacterium tuberculosis* or human immunodeficiency virus (HIV), or an acute illness followed by complete recovery as in most cases of influenza, hepatitis A or leishmania infection, or even subclinical infection.

Mechanisms of evasion

The evolution of a successful parasite pitted against the evolution of the mammalian adaptive immune response has been described as 'a game of chess played over millennia'. Figure 11.2 pinpoints 22 mechanisms by which pathogens have been shown to evade the defensive activity of the immune system. These are described in more detail below. Some of the more successful pathogens have developed multiple mechanisms of evasion, e.g. the more virulent staphylococci and streptococci, mycobacteria, herpes simplex virus and HIV, malarial parasites, schistosomes and trypanosomes. With some infections, the battle is such that variation in the ability of the individual host to mount an effective response leads to a clinical spectrum of disease ranging from chronic and sometimes overwhelming infection to containment or destruction of the parasite and heightened immunity (e.g. lepromatous vs. tuberculoid leprosy). The immune response to larger parasites rarely eliminates the organism completely. In some protozoan infections (e.g. malaria) immunity to reinfection is only present when the initial infection persists (known as 'premunition' or non-sterile immunity) and in helminth infections (e.g. schistosomiasis) adult worms survive but reinfection with larval forms is resisted ('concomitant immunity').

EXAMPLES OF EVASIVE MECHANISMS (See Fig. 11.2)

1. Sequestration. Wart papilloma virus in the outer epidermis, staphylococci in bone (osteomyelitis), herpes simplex virus in sensory neurones, tapeworms in hydatid cysts and retroviruses (e.g. HIV) integrated into host DNA are inaccessible to the immune response.

2. Disguise. Schistosomes cover their surface with various host proteins, e.g. blood group substances and HLA proteins.

3. Antigenic variation. The parasites that cause African trypanosomiasis possess genes that code for about 1000 variant forms of their surface glycoproteins; malarial parasites also display a number of surface variants, and longer term changes in influenza virus surface proteins (i.e. haemagglutinin and neuraminidase) mean that immunity is rarely sustained.

4. Antigen shedding. Organisms that shed surface antigens in abundance, e.g. *Streptococcus pneumoniae, Plasmodium falciparum* and *Schistosoma mansoni*, can neutralize the antibody response at a distance.

5. Resistance to complement. Bacteria with well-developed capsules (e.g. those containing sialic acid) are able to resist the effects of complement activation by enhancing the action of complement inhibitors (e.g. H and I) or by preventing interaction between fixed C3b and C3 receptors on phagocytes. Examples include *Haemophilus influenzae, Staphylococcus aureus,* and *Strep. pneumoniae.*

6. Cleavage of immunoglobulin molecules. Several bacteria that gain access via mucosal surfaces (i.e. *Neisseria gonorrhoeae, Strep. pneumoniae* and *H. influenzae*) have a protease that cleaves IgA molecules into Fab and Fc portions. A similar activity has been demonstrated with *Trypanosoma cruzi.* This process has been called 'fabulation'.

7. Fc binding. Herpes simplex virus, varicella-zoster virus and some staphylococci produce a protein that binds to the Fc fragment of IgG, and some streptococci produce a substance that binds to the Fc of IgA. This inhibits the ability of the Fc fragment to opsonize or activate complement.

8. *Inactivation of complement.* Herpes simplex virus has a glycoprotein (gC) that binds C3b; *Pseudomonas aeruginosa* has an elastase that inactivates C3b and C5a, and leishmania organisms are able to eject membrane attack complexes from their cell membrane.

9. *Inhibition of attachment.* Some organisms, e.g. *Toxoplasma gondi*, are able to inhibit attachment to the phagocyte surface but the chemical basis for this phenomenon is not understood.

10. *Inhibition of phagocytosis.* Several organisms can resist phagocytosis due to the properties of their surface coat or capsule, e.g. *Strep. pneumoniae*, *Candida albicans* and African trypanosomes.

11. *Inhibition of chemotaxis.* The process by which phagocytes are attracted into sites of inflammation is inhibited by several organisms, e.g. *Clostridium perfringens*, *Staph. aureus* and some streptococci.

12. *Blocking access of cells.* Some staphylococci liberate a coagulase which causes fibrin deposition and blocks access to inflammatory cells.

13. *Phagocyte toxicity.* Some organisms have a toxic effect on phagocytes. Staphylococcal leucocidins and streptococcal haemolysins disrupt polymorph granules and release enzymes into the cytoplasm, and some chlamydial organisms have a similar effect on macrophages. *Bordetella pertussis* releases a toxin resembling adenyl cyclase which arrests the phagocytic process, and some organisms (e.g. *Bacillus anthracis*) lyse the phagocyte on direct contact.

14. *Escape from the phagosome.* Mycobacterium leprae and T. cruzi enter the phagosome but then escape from it into the cytoplasm.

15. *Resistance to killing.* Some organisms possess cell walls that resist oxidative killing, e.g. *Mycobacterium tuberculosis*, *Yersinia pestis*, *Brucella abortus* and *B. anthracis*. Some staphylococci produce catalase and can inhibit hydrogen peroxide. Leishmania produce a superoxide dismutase and have an anti-oxidant effect.

16. *Inhibition of phagosome–lysosome fusion.* Several organisms, e.g. *M. tuberculosis*, *T. gondi* and legionella organisms are able to inhibit the process of phagosome–lysosome fusion but the biochemical mechanism is unclear.

17. *Resistance to digestion.* Encapsulated organisms, e.g. *H. influenzae*, and *Strep. pneumoniae* can resist lysosomal digestion. Some leishmania produce a lysosomal enzyme inhibitor (gp63).

18. *Impairment of the interferon response.* The interferon response is compromised by leishmania organisms and by hepatitis B virus. Epstein–Barr virus produces a molecule (BCRFI) resembling IL-10 which inhibits IFN-γ synthesis in T cells and LGL.

19. *Inhibition of cytokines.* Cytokines (e.g. IL-2 and TNF) can be inhibited by some pathogens (e.g. *T. cruzi*).

20. *Lymphocyte activation.* Quite a few organisms, e.g. staphylococci, plasmodia, trypanosomes and Epstein–Barr virus, have been shown to activate lymphocytes polyclonally. In some instances this effect is mediated by 'superantigens' (e.g. staphylococcal enterotoxin) that bind to a broad spectrum of T cell receptors. This can prevent a specific response to the pathogen.

21. *Lymphocyte suppression.* Immunosuppression is a feature of several severe infections, e.g. measles, malaria, lepromatous leprosy and HIV infection. The mechanisms of helper T cell depletion in HIV infection are discussed on p. 170.

22. *HLA expression.* Several viruses that are able to establish latent or persistent infections e.g. adenovirus, cytomegalovirus and herpes simplex virus (HSV), have been shown to inhibit HLA class I surface expression. In the case of HSV this is achieved by the production of a protein that binds to the peptide transporter protein (see p. 51) and blocks the presentation of viral peptides to cytotoxic T cells.

The inflammatory response

Pathogens are ultimately destroyed by extracellular lysis or intracellular digestion but a series of amplifying events is required to ensure that all the relevant cells and molecules arrive at the right place at the right time.

DISSEMINATION OF THE IMMUNE RESPONSE

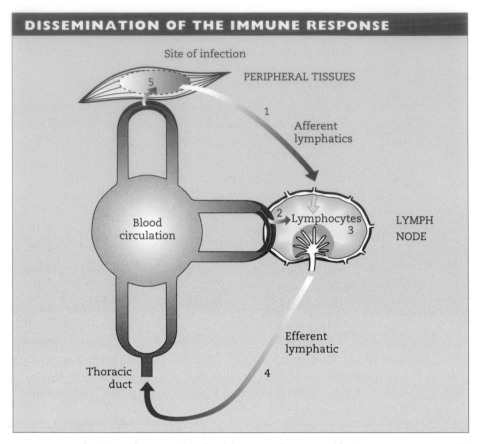

Fig. 11.3 The steps involved in mounting a specific immune response. (1) Antigen (both free and on antigen presenting cells) is transported from the site of infection to the draining lymph node; (2) lymphocytes enter the node from the blood across high endothelial venules; (3) activation of antigen-specific lymphocytes; (4) activated lymphocytes enter the circulation; (5) cells and mediators (e.g. lymphocytes, macrophages, granulocytes, antibodies and complement) pass across activated endothelium into the site of infection.

This involves a modification of the normal recirculation of lymphocytes, discussed in Chapter 4 (Fig. 4.7), to ensure that lymphocytes specific for the antigens of the invading organism are optimally activated and are targeted to the site of infection (Fig. 11.3). The secondary lymphoid tissues (e.g. lymph nodes) draining the infected tissues provide the optimal environment for interaction between antigens, antigen presenting cells and recirculating lymphocytes, leading to the activation of specific T and B cells (discussed in Chapter 4). The recruitment of specific lymphocytes and antibodies, as well as other defensive cells and molecules, to the site of infection involves inflammatory changes in the infected tissues,

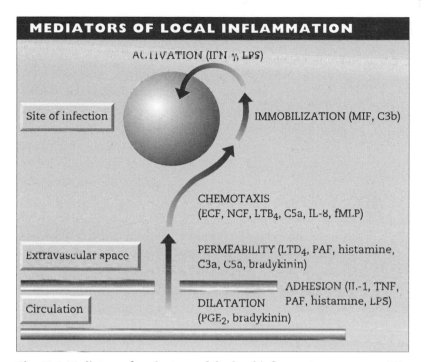

Fig. 11.4 Mediators of each stage of the local inflammatory response. PG, prostaglandin; IL, interleukin; TNF, tumour necrosis factor; PAF, platelet activating factor; LPS, lipopolysaccharide; LT, leukotriene; ECF, eosinophil chemotactic factor; NCF, neutrophil chemotactic factor; fMLP, formyl-methionyl-leucyl phenylalanine; MIF, migration inhibition factor; IFN, interferon.

particularly affecting the blood vessels which provide the route of entry to the site (Fig. 11.3). These events include **vasodilatation, adhesion of** leucocytes to endothelium, increased vascular **permeability**, the chemical attraction of inflammatory cells, i.e. **chemotaxis, immobilization** of cells at the site of inflammation, and **activation** of the relevant cells and molecules to liberate their lytic products (see Fig. 11.4). The clinical signs of inflammation, i e rubor (erythema), tumor (swelling), calor (heat) and dolor (pain) were described by Celsus almost 2000 years ago.

THE MOLECULAR BASIS OF TISSUE INFLAMMATION

The variety of chemical mediators which promote each stage of inflammation are indicated in Fig. 11.4. These are variously derived from lymphocytes, mast cells, other leucocytes and tissue cells, complement and other serum proteins, and even microbes themselves. The apparent redundancy of several mediators exerting similar effects (Table 11.4) ensures the efficacy of the response in different types or sites of infection.

It is at sites of infection that circulating leucocytes employ cell surface

adhesion molecules to bind to vascular endothelium and migrate into the underlying tissues (Fig. 11.5). These inflammatory processes are similar to those involved in the homing of lymphocytes to secondary lymphoid tissues during normal lymphocyte recirculation (p. 59, Fig. 4.7). Inflammatory mediators induce vascular endothelial cells to express adhesion molecules called **selectins** (P-selectin and E-selectin) which interact with heavily glycosylated proteins called **mucins** on the surface of leucocytes. Conversely, leucocytes express L-selectin which binds to endothelial mucins. These interactions are responsible for the initial capture of a circulating leucocyte, which then rolls along the blood vessel wall. Cytokines stimulate the endothelial cells to express other **cell adhesion molecules (CAM)** ICAM-1 and VCAM-1 which are ligands for the **integrins** LFA-1 and VLA-4 respectively. Inflammatory mediators activate these integrins on the captured leucocytes, resulting in strong adhesion to the underlying endothelium. The leucocytes then migrate between endothelial cell junctions; secrete enzymes to digest the vascular basement membrane, and migrate towards the site of infection in response to chemotactic mediators emanating from that site.

THE SYSTEMIC RESPONSE TO INFECTION

These defensive processes operating at local level are supported by systemic responses that enhance their effectiveness; limit tissue damage,

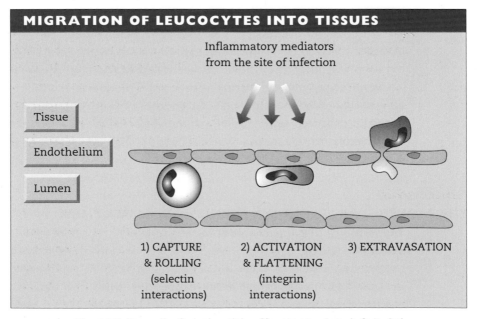

Fig. 11.5 Stages in the migration of leucocytes into infected tissues.

THE INFLAMMATORY RESPONSE

Effect	Mediating cytokines			Site of action
	IL-1	IL-6	TNF	
Fever	+	+	+	Hypothalamus
Leucocytosis	+	+		Bone marrow
Acute phase	+	+	+	Liver
Glucocorticoid release	+	+		Pituitary and adrenal

Table 11.5 Coordination of the inflammatory response.

and promote healing. These consist of fever, leucocytosis, acute phase protein production and glucocorticoid release, and form part of the coordinated inflammatory response mediated by the cytokines IL-1, IL-6 and TNF (Table 11.5). These cytokines are released mostly from macrophages and lymphocytes and act locally on lymphocytes which release other cytokines (e.g. IL-2 and IL-4), mediate cytotoxicity and synthesize antibody. Cytokines also activate neutrophils, and induce the expression of HLA glycoproteins and adhesion molecules on endothelial and other cells.

Fever

Fever is a prominent feature of many infections but can be severe, e.g. in malaria, pneumonia and septicaemia, or prolonged, e.g. in brucellosis, osteomyelitis and tuberculosis. The existence of an 'endogenous pyrogen' had been known for many years but this activity is now attributed to the cytokines, IL-1, IL-6, TNF and, possibly, Interferon. These act on the thermoregulatory centre in the hypothalamus via production of the prostaglandin PGE_2. The resultant rise in body temperature enhances various cellular and biochemical processes, e.g. the bactericidal activity of polymorphs, antiviral effects of interferon, proliferative responses of lymphocytes and antibody production.

Leucocytosis

Many infections are associated with an increase in the number of polymorphonuclear leucocytes (**leucocytosis**) or lymphocytes (**lymphocytosis**) in the circulation. This is mediated by IL-1 and IL-6 and the production of colony stimulating factors specific for these cell types. The rapid release of less mature polymorphonuclear cells from bone marrow gives rise to a preponderance of cells in peripheral blood which lack the nuclear hypersegmentation characteristic of mature neutrophils (often referred to as a 'left shift'). In severe or prolonged infection, the neutrophil azurophilic lysosomal granules stain more readily and give an appearance which has been called 'toxic granulation' although it is largely due to increased enzyme activity.

The acute phase response

A number of plasma proteins that have roles in inflammation or the healing process are produced in increased amounts by the liver during infection and after injury. This effect is mediated by the action of IL-1, IL-6 and TNF on hepatocytes. Human acute phase proteins can be subdivided into groups according to the magnitude of their increase (Table 11.6). Those with the shortest response time show the highest increases in concentration. Acute phase reactants operate as mediators, inhibitors or scavengers of cell-derived products. **C-reactive protein** binds to phosphorylcholine and several other molecules present on the surface of some microorganisms (e.g. *Strep. pneumoniae*). Bound CRP activates the classical complement pathway and may have an immunomodulatory effect. The α_1-**acid glycoprotein** also has inhibitory effects. Some acute phase proteins act as enzyme inhibitors: α_1-**antitrypsin** inhibits neutral proteases (e.g. collagenase and elastase), α_1-**antichymotrypsin** inhibits cathepsin G, and **haptoglobin** inhibits other lysosomal cathepsins. Haptoglobin also conserves the iron released from haemoglobin during inflammation and serum amyloid A protein helps to clear cholesterol

ACUTE PHASE PROTEINS

Protein	Plasma concentration (g l⁻¹)		Response time (h)
	Normal	In inflammation	
C-reactive protein	c. 0.0005	0.4	6–10
Serum amyloid A protein	c. 0.005	2.5	6–10
α_1-Antichymotrypsin	c. 0.5	3.0	10
α_1-Antitrypsin	c. 1.5	7.0	
α_1-Acid glycoprotein	c. 1.0	3.0	24
Haptoglobin	c. 2.0	6.0	
Fibrinogen	c. 3.0	10.0	
Caeruloplasmin	c. 0.5	2.0	
C3	c. 1.0	3.0	48–72
C4	c. 0.3	1.0	

Table 11.6 Human acute phase proteins. (After Whicher & Evans 1992.)

accumulated during the phagocytosis of cell debris. **Caeruloplasmin** is a scavenger of superoxide radicals and prevents the auto-oxidation of lipids.

Glucocorticoid release

IL-1 and IL-6 interact with the hypothalamic–pituitary–adrenal axis at two levels: in the hypothalamus they induce the production of corticotrophin releasing factor which mediates adrenocorticotrophic hormone (ACTH) release, and they also act directly on the adrenal cortex both of which result in the release of anti-inflammatory **glucocorticoids** (e.g. cortisol). This is a key part of the systemic response to trauma and infection and limits the destructive effects of inflammation.

Regulation of immune and inflammatory responses

The cells and molecules of the immune system possess considerable destructive potential which, if unleashed inappropriately, can inflict fatal effects on host tissues. It is, therefore, essential that immune responses to foreign pathogens are strictly regulated in magnitude and duration. This is achieved by a range of inhibitory factors, some examples of which are given in Table 11.7.

REGULATORS OF INFLAMMATION

Inhibited components	Inhibitors
T cells	Transforming growth factor-β Interleukin-4 and interleukin-10 (inhibit T_H1 cells) Interferon-γ (inhibits T_H2 cells)
Cytokines	Interleukin-1 receptor antagonist (competes for receptor binding) Soluble cytokine receptors (prevent binding to cell surface receptors)
Mast cell mediators	Histaminase and aryl sulphatase (from eosinophils)
Complement	C1 esterase inhibitor Decay accelerating factor Complement receptor-1 Membrane cofactor protein Factor H Factor I

Table 11.7 Regulators of immune and inflammatory activity.

Diagnosis of microbial infection

Infection with most bacteria and some other organisms is usually diagnosed by laboratory culture; characterization of the organism's biochemical properties, inhibitory or toxic effects, and analysis of its antigenic structure or susceptibility to other agents (e.g. bacteriophages and antibiotics). Light or electron microscopy is preferred for some organisms in view of its speed and the characteristic appearance of some organisms. The detection of free antigen in body fluids or tissues offers advantages in some infections and usually involves the use of techniques such as agglutination, immunofluorescence, ELISA or RIA methods (see Chapter 6). Nucleic acid hybridization *in situ* or involving the polymerase chain reaction (PCR) are other means by which infection can be diagnosed without culture of the organism (Table 11.8).

Many infections are diagnosed serologically, i.e. by the identification of specific antibody in serum or other body fluids (e.g. saliva). This involves the use of techniques such as complement fixation, neutralization, agglutination inhibition, immunofluorescence, immunoperoxidase, ELISA or RIA (see Chapter 6). Skin testing is still used to measure the immune response in some circumstances, e.g. the tuberculin test for tuberculosis.

Opportunistic infection

Some individuals are especially prone to infection with recognized pathogens or may be susceptible to infection with less virulent organisms that do not cause disease in normal individuals. These so-called **opportunistic infections** are a not infrequent sequel to many of the procedures involved in modern medical care in which host defences may be bypassed or treatments given which have immunosuppressive effects (Table 11.9).

DIAGNOSIS OF MICROBIAL INFECTION
Light or electron microscopy
Culture and identification
Antigen detection
Nucleotide analysis
Serology
Skin testing

Table 11.8 The diagnosis of microbial infection.

CONDITIONS FAVOURING OPPORTUNISTIC INFECTION

Bypassing host defences	Burns and other trauma
	Eczema
	Invasive procedures e.g., intravenous lines and other indwelling devices
Primary immunodeficiency disorders	(see Chapter 13)
Diseases causing impaired immunity	Infections e.g. malaria, leprosy, AIDS
	Chronic inflammatory disease, e.g. systemic lupus
	Lymphoproliferative disease, e.g. chronic lymphatic leukaemia, Hodgkin's disease, myelomatosis
	Metabolic disorders, e.g. diabetes, uraemia
	Malnutrition
	Protein-losing states
	Prematurity and old age
Treatment leading to impaired immunity	Immunosuppressive drugs or other forms of lymphoid ablation used in the management of haematological, chronic inflammatory and malignant diseases, and transplantation

Table 11.9 Examples of conditions which favour opportunistic infection.

The possibility of impaired immunity should always be considered when infections occur unusually frequently, in unusual locations, or are due to unusual organisms. The pattern of infection often points to the nature of the underlying defect (see Chapter 13 & Tables 13.1 & 13.9). Various diseases cause impaired immunity, e.g. chronic lymphatic leukaemia, nephrotic syndrome, uraemia, chronic infection and malnutrition (see Tables 11.9 & 13.8).

Most immunosuppressive drugs inhibit T cell responses and their use may be complicated by opportunistic infection with enveloped viruses, intracellular bacteria and protozoa (see Table 18.2). Patients with severe neutropenia (i.e. having a peripheral blood leucocyte count of $< 500\,mm^{-3}$) pose a special problem as the absence of a normal inflammatory response makes it difficult to diagnose acute infection. Here, as for many other patients with impaired defences, it is often necessary to perform microbiological screening and administer the most relevant form of antimicrobial therapy on an empirical basis. Patients who are unduly prone to opportunistic infection for long periods (e.g. after bone marrow transplantation) may require protective isolation in special units.

Chronic inflammatory diseases of unknown cause

There are a number of chronic and often severe diseases which, although they show abundant evidence of immunological stimulation have yet to be associated with an infective agent. Examples include: rheumatoid arthritis, sarcoidosis, ulcerative colitis, type 1 diabetes, chronic hepatitis, various forms of glomerulonephritis and multiple sclerosis. Most of them are slow in their evolution and show a characteristic pattern of genetic susceptibility linked to HLA Class II loci (see Chapter 16). The development of diagnostic techniques that do not depend on culture of the organism (e.g. PCR), combined with advances in epidemiology, is beginning to point to microbial causes for some of these conditions. This should lead to preventive measures for these diseases as they are often resistant to treatment once they have become established.

The host:pathogen interface

The outcome of a particular infection depends on many factors which govern the ability of the pathogen to invade, evade and damage the host and the ability of the immune response to recognize and destroy the pathogen. Any weakening of the pathogen (often achieved by the administration of **antimicrobial chemotherapy**) or strengthening of the specific immune response against it (e.g. by **immunization**) will favour the immune response whereas successful **evasion** by the parasite or the development of **immunodeficiency** (be it inherited or acquired) will tip the scales in favour of the pathogen (Fig. 11.6).

It is not surprising that the outcome for the host is often 'survival at a price' and that damage to host tissues is a common finding during the course of most infectious diseases. The pathological consequences of the

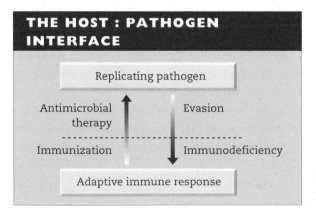

Fig. 11.6 The host:pathogen interface and factors which affect it.

endeavours of the immune response during its response to foreign material are referred to as **hypersensitivity** (in the course of an infection), **allergy** (when the trigger is inanimate) and **autoimmunity**, when the response is directed at self. These phenomena are described in more detail in Chapters 14–16.

KEY POINTS

1 Infectious diseases are still a major threat to life and health throughout the world even though the popular impression in the West until recently was that scourges of infection were a thing of the past. Tuberculosis, malaria and HIV infection are just three examples of infectious diseases that each threaten the lives of tens of millions of individuals.

2 The complexity of the immune response and its multiplicity of mechanisms for destroying infectious agents reflect the many ways that pathogens have developed to evade the attentions of the immune response. Twenty-two examples of these mechanisms are cited in this chapter and set against a summary of the sequential layers of host defence.

3 The inflammatory response augments the actions of the immune system. At local level, this consists of enhanced vascular adhesiveness and permeability, associated with chemotaxis, immobilization, and activation of inflammatory cells. Systemically, this is supported by the production of fever, leucocytosis, acute phase proteins and the release of glucocorticoids which are together mediated by IL-1, IL 6 and TNF released from macrophages and lymphocytes. Regulation of these processes is necessary to avoid excessive damage to host tissues.

4 Traditionally, infections have been diagnosed by culturing organisms in the laboratory from clinical samples. Increasingly, these techniques are being augmented or replaced by other methods for the detection of chemical sequences – often nucleotides – that are specific for particular groups or species of organisms, and methods that characterize the antibody response to infecting organisms. These approaches are proving of particular value in many of the chronic immunological diseases that are triggered by microbes but which do not yield culturable microbes in clinical samples.

Further reading

Adams D.H. & Shaw S. (1994) Leucocyte–endothelial interactions and regulation of leucocyte migration. *Lancet*, **343**, 831–836.

Banatvala N. & Feldman R. (1993) The epidemiology of *Helicobacter pylori*: missing pieces in a jigsaw. *Communicable Disease Report*, **3**, R56–59.

Bloom B.R. & Murray C.J.L. (1992) Tuberculosis: commentary on a reemergent killer. *Science*, **257**, 1055–1064.

Duerden B.I., Reid T.M.S. & Jewsbury J.M. (1993) *Microbial and Parasitic Infection*. Edward Arnold, London.

Krause R.M. (1992) The origin of plagues: Old and New. *Science*, **257**, 1073–1078.

Lederberg J., Shope R.E. & Oaks S.C. eds. (1992) *Emerging Infections: Microbial Threats to Health in the United States*. National Academy Press, Washington DC.

Mims C.A. (1995) *The Pathogenesis of Infectious Disease*, 4th edn. Academic Press London.

Norden C.W. & Kuller L.H. (1984) Identifying infectious etiologies of chronic disease. *Review of Infectious Diseases*, **6**, 200–213.

Paul W.E. (1994) Infectious diseases and the immune system. In *Life, Death and the Immune System: Scientific American: A Special Issue*. W.H. Freeman, New York.

Saboor S.A., Johnson N.McI. & McFadden J. (1992) Detection of mycobacterial DNA in sarcoidosis and tuberculosis with polymerase chain reaction. *Lancet*, **339**, 1012–1015.

Sissons J.G.P., Borysiewicz L.K. & Cohen J. eds (1994) *Immunology of Infection*. Kluwer Academic, London.

Springer T.A. (1994) Traffic signals for lymphocyte recirculation and leukocyte emigration: the multistep paradigm. *Cell*, **76**, 301–314.

Teo C.G. (1992) The virology and serology of hepatitis: an overview. *Communicable Disease Report*, **2**, R109–R114.

Warren K.S. ed. (1993) *Immunology and Molecular Biology of Parasitic Infections*, 3rd edn. Blackwell Scientific Publications, Oxford.

Whicher J.T. & Evans S.W. eds. (1992) *Biochemistry of Inflammation*. Kluwer Academic, London.

CHAPTER 12

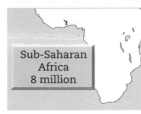

Sub-Saharan
Africa
8 million

HIV Infection
and AIDS

The acquired immunodeficiency syndrome (AIDS) has been a major preoccupation of the lay and scientific media since it burst upon the scene in 1981. Study of the slow but relentless decay of the immune system and the pattern of infections that characterize this condition has highlighted the importance of immunology in health and disease. Public perceptions and expert assessments of the prospects for preventing, or even curing, this otherwise fatal condition have fluctuated widely but the challenge has already stimulated many innovations in basic science, laboratory diagnosis, drug and vaccine development, and approaches to patient care.

The chronology listed in Table 12.1 outlines the progress made in identifying the causative virus, in developing serological testing, and the introduction of antiviral agents. It has recently become clear, however, that zidovudine (azidothymidine) has little impact on the natural history of the disease and it is hoped that combination chemotherapy and the development of vaccines will prove more effective.

Clinical features

Those who become infected usually remain asymptomatic for many years, although 10–15 per cent experience a febrile illness resembling infectious mononucleosis around the time when HIV antibody first becomes detectable (seroconversion). Later on, there may be persistent lymph node swelling (lymphadenopathy) without other symptoms. The addition of weight loss, fever, diarrhoea and minor opportunistic infections (e.g. oral candidiasis, herpes zoster or tuberculosis) constitutes the **AIDS-related complex (ARC)** and the case definition for **AIDS** is fulfilled when more severe opportunistic infections (e.g. *Pneumocystis carinii* pneumonia, toxoplasmosis, cryptococcosis or cytomegalovirus infection) or tumours (e.g. lymphoma or Kaposi's sarcoma) supervene.

HISTORICAL SEQUENCE OF EVENTS

Event	Year
First description of AIDS	1981
Discovery of HIV	1983
HIV antibody testing introduced	1985
Zidovudine (azidothymidine) approved for clinical use	1987
Start of vaccine trials in uninfected volunteers	1990

Table 12.1 Historical sequence of events.

Table 12.2 lists the infections to which these patients are prone. The peripheral blood CD4$^+$ T cell count declines progressively during the symptomatic phase of the illness, the more severe infections occurring when the CD4 count has fallen below 200 cells mm^{-3}. The mean incubation period from infection to the development of AIDS is 8–10 years in industrialized countries but survival times are often reduced in the developing world where death may follow less severe opportunistic infections.

Epidemiology

AIDS was first recognized among male homosexuals in California and New York but cases were soon documented throughout Europe and in sub-Saharan Africa, and have since been identified in almost every country in the world. In Africa, transmission is mostly via heterosexual contact and the number of male and female cases is almost equal. Most European cases have been attributed to infection acquired through sexual intercourse between men but the proportion infected by heterosexual contact has risen steeply in recent years. The human immunodeficiency virus (HIV) is transmitted by similar routes to hepatitis B virus but has lower infectivity. The major routes are unprotected sexual intercourse, infected blood or blood products, injecting drug use, or from mother to infant. The introduction of antibody screening for HIV infection in many industrialized countries has enabled fairly precise estimates to be made of the incidence and prevalence of infection. However, the long latent period before AIDS develops has led to gross underestimates of the prevalence of HIV infection in many developing countries that have not been able to introduce serological surveillance until recently, e.g. India and Thailand. The incidence curve for AIDS cases in the UK has stabilized at about 1500 new cases per year although those cases in which infection was

INFECTIONS OCCURRING IN AIDS	
Organism	**Site of infection**
Viruses	
Herpes simplex	Skin, oropharynx
Varicella-zoster	Skin
Cytomegalovirus	Gut, lung, retina
Polyoma (JC) virus	Central nervous system
Bacteria	
M. tuberculosis	Lung
M. avium intracellulare	Disseminated
Salmonella species	Gut
Rochalimea species	Skin, liver, central nervous system
Protozoa	
Toxoplasma gondii	Central nervous system
Cryptosporidium species	Gut
Giardia lamblia	Gut
Isospora belli	Gut
Pneumocystis carinii	Lung
Fungi	
Candida albicans	Oropharynx, oesophagus
Cryptococcus neoformans	Central nervous system
Coccidiodes immitis	Disseminated
Histoplasma capsulatum	Disseminated
Nematodes	
Strongyloides stercoralis	Gut

Table 12.2 The spectrum of infection in AIDS.

acquired heterosexually (currently almost 300 annually) continue to increase in number. The World Health Organization (WHO) has estimated that over 3 million cases of AIDS had occurred worldwide by late 1993 and that the number of people with HIV infection will rise toward 40 million by the year 2000. More than 90 per cent of these cases will occur in developing countries (Fig. 12.1).

Virology

Only two closely related retroviruses, HIV 1 and HIV 2, have been shown to cause AIDS in man despite much speculation to the contrary. HIV 2

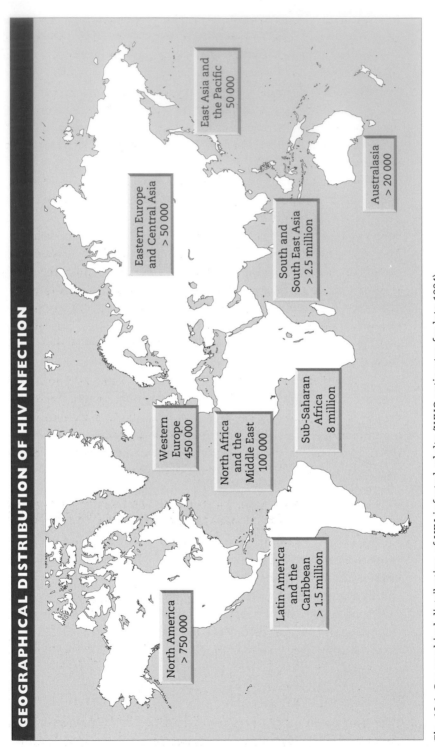

Fig. 12.1 Geographical distribution of HIV-infected adults (WHO estimates for late 1994).

infection is rare outside West Africa but both viruses are thought to have originated from a related primate virus. Several other retroviruses are known to cause immunodeficiency syndromes in other mammals, e.g. feline immunodeficiency virus in cats and simian immunodeficiency virus in macaques. Visna-maedi virus affects sheep and causes wasting and neurological features resembling those seen in AIDS but without immunodeficiency. Human T lymphotropic viruses I and II are also transmitted by blood but cause leukaemia or neurological disease without immunodeficiency.

HIV has a strong affinity for the helper T cell. This is mediated by several of its structural components (Table 12.3). The major envelope glycoprotein (gp120) binds to the CD4 receptor and an associated glycoprotein (gp41) promotes fusion with the lymphocyte membrane. The virus also contains an RNA polymerase (to enable it to synthesize DNA), other enzymes, and structural and regulatory proteins. Considerable variation occurs in the biochemical structure of the major envelope protein during the course of an infection. HIV nucleotide sequences are detectable in about 1 in 10 000 CD4$^+$ T cells during asymptomatic infection but the frequency rises to 1 in 100 cells when AIDS develops.

Kaposi's sarcoma is more common in patients with AIDS who have acquired their infection sexually compared with those who have contracted it via infected blood or blood products. It is rarely seen in association with other immunodeficiency disorders and molecular microbiological techniques have recently demonstrated the presence of a new human herpes virus (HHV8) in patients with Kaposi's sarcoma.

COMPONENTS OF HIV

Genes	Products
Structural	
ENV	gp160 (gp120 + gp41)
GAG	Core proteins (p24, p17, p15)
Enzymes	
POL	Reverse transcriptase, protease, integrase, ribonuclease
Regulatory	
TAT	
REV	Activating and regulatory proteins
NEF	

Table 12.3 Principal components of HIV.

LABORATORY DIAGNOSIS

Currently, this is usually achieved by the detection of antibody to HIV using an ELISA screening test followed by a confirmatory Western blot. Detection of the virus itself is still largely a research procedure although the polymerase chain reaction can be used to detect HIV-specific nucleotide sequences in clinical specimens. Recent work suggests that some patients exposed to HIV may show evidence of a T cell response to the virus but remain seronegative for antibody. The balance between T cell and B cell responsiveness (and the outcome of infection) is likely to be determined by the dose and route by which HIV gains access and it has been proposed that a strong T_H1 response may be protective in contrast to a T_H2 response which favours antibody production (see p. 46).

Immunology

In cases of HIV infection defined by seropositivity, antibodies to the envelope (gp120, gp41) or core (p24) proteins are usually detectable within 1–3 months of exposure. Detectable core antigen has usually disappeared by the time antibody develops. The level of core antibody falls as the disease progresses toward AIDS when the CD4 lymphocyte count falls below 500 cells mm^{-3} and opportunistic infections occur.

The cause of the progressive immunodeficiency that characterizes AIDS is poorly understood but there are several possibilities (Table 12.4). The virus may have a direct lytic action on the CD4$^+$ T cell although little free HIV is detectable after the initial brief viraemic phase. However, the combination of CD4 attachment and fusion mediated by the envelope proteins (gp120 and gp41) leads to the formation of multinuclear aggregates of T cells often referred to as syncytia. This, and the internalization of CD4–gp160 complexes, has adverse effects on T cell function. The immune response directed to HIV-infected helper T cells may be mediated by antibody-dependent mechanisms (e.g. ADCC or complement-mediated cytotoxicity) or by the CD8$^+$ cytotoxic T cell and in each case is likely to impair T cell function in general.

MECHANISMS OF T CELL DEPLETION

Virus-induced lysis
Syncytia formation
Immune lysis (by antibody or cellular
  mechanisms)
Induction of apoptosis

Table 12.4 Possible mechanisms of helper T cell depletion in HIV infection.

The process of **apoptosis** or programmed cell death is the mechanism by which self-reactive T cells are eliminated during T cell differentiation in the thymus (see p. 44). Mature T cells usually respond to receptor stimulation by cytokine secretion and proliferation but T cells taken from patients with HIV infection develop apoptosis when subjected to stimuli that would normally result in their activation. It is not known how this abnormal signal is generated but the binding of gp120 to CD4 receptors and their cross-linking by antibody to the envelope protein are likely to subvert the helper T cell's response to antigenic stimulation.

The ability of HIV to infect antigen presenting cells, e.g. dendritic cells and macrophages, may also impair the immune response and, by altering the pattern of cytokine secretion, may affect the balance between type 1 and type 2 helper T cell responses and cell-mediated vs. antibody dominance. The succession of antigenic variants of HIV that develops during the course of an infection also militates against the success of the immune response and some strains may be more effective in inducing immunosuppression.

Management

The stage of infection at which the CD4$^+$ lymphocyte count falls below 500 cells mm^{-3} and opportunistic infections develop is usually the point at which treatment with antiviral agents is commenced. The reverse transcriptase inhibitor, azidothymidine (AZT) has been the drug of choice for several years but it has toxic effects on the bone marrow, liver and kidneys. Other nucleoside analogues, e.g. di-deoxyinosine (DDI) and di-deoxycytidine (DDC) are also being evaluated but although each produce some benefit they also have toxic side effects. Recent trials suggest that introducing AZT during the asymptomatic stage of HIV infection does not delay progression to AIDS. Prophylactic treatment for *Pneumocystis carinii* infection is usually introduced when the CD4 lymphocyte count falls below 200 cells mm^{-3} and other opportunistic infections are treated as they arise.

Prevention

Public health measures and health education programmes can be effective in reducing the risk of infection by promoting safer sexual practices, by encouraging the prompt treatment of other sexually transmitted diseases, by reducing the opportunity for injecting drug users to share needles, and the provision of safe blood for transfusion and preparation of blood products.

However, control of the global epidemic of HIV infection will not be possible until an effective means of curing or preventing the disease becomes available. Considerable enterprise has been directed toward the development of an effective vaccine. Safety and immunogenicity studies have been completed for several vaccines most of which contain part or all of the envelope protein. Larger scale efficacy trials in uninfected groups with a high risk of infection are planned to take place in Africa, Asia and South America.

KEY POINTS

1 Considerable advances have been made since HIV infection was first observed in 1981, including the identification of the causative virus, the application of HIV antibody testing, the introduction of antiviral agents, and the start of vaccine trials. However, there is still no effective treatment for this infection which gradually overwhelms the immune system of an individual over a period of 10 years or so.

2 It is transmitted by sexual intercourse, infected blood or blood products, injecting drug use or from infected mother to infant. The WHO estimates that there will be 40 million cases of infection by the year 2000, with 90 per cent of them occurring in developing countries.

3 HIV binds to the CD4 receptor on T helper cells and the peripheral blood CD4 lymphocyte count declines progressively. Opportunistic infections with other organisms develop when the count falls below 400 cells mm^{-3} and become severe when it falls below 200 cells mm^{-3}.

4 The diagnosis is usually made by detecting specific antibody using ELISA and Western blot methods but the balance between T and B cell responsiveness may determine whether or not a patient becomes positive for antibody following infection.

5 The decline in T cell function is likely to be due to some or all of the following mechanisms: direct viral lysis, the fusion of lymphocytes by the formation of syncitia, immunological destruction of the infected cells, and the induction of apoptosis.

6 Much can be done to treat opportunistic infections but the main prospect for successful intervention is the development of an effective vaccine. Trials are in progress but it is unlikely that this will be swiftly achieved.

7 In the meantime, public health measures are the only means of slowing the spread of infection in communities. These include: safe sexual practices, prompt treatment of other sexually transmitted diseases, preventing drug users sharing needles, and providing safe blood and blood products.

Further reading

Ada G. (1993) Towards phase III trials for candidate vaccines. *Nature*, **364**, 489–490.

Greene W.C. (1993) AIDS and the immune system. *Scientific American*, **269**, 67–73.

Levy J.A. (1995) A new human herpesvirus: KSHV or HHV8? *Lancet*, **346**, 786.

McCarthy G.A. & Mercey D. (1994) The changing clinical features of HIV-1 infection in the United Kingdom. *Communicable Disease Report*, **4**, R53–R58.

Pinching A.J. (1993) Clinical aspects of AIDS and HIV infection. In Lachmann P.J., Peters D.K., Rosen F.S. & Walport M.J. eds, *Clinical Aspects of Immunology*, 5th edn. Blackwell Scientific Publications, Oxford.

Rowland-Jones S.L. & McMichael A. (1995) Immune responses in HIV-exposed seronegatives: have they repelled the virus? *Current Opinion in Immunology*, **7**, 448–455.

Weiss R.A. (1993) How does HIV cause AIDS? *Science*, **260**, 1273–1279.

WHO (1995) WHO AIDS data at 31 December 1994 and the current global situation of the HIV/AIDS pandemic. *Weekly Epidemiological Record*, **70**, 5–8.

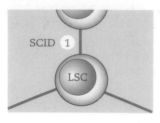

Immunodeficiency Disorders

The immune system and the complex interrelationships of its components have evolved to cope with the enormous variety of pathogens which threaten the host organism. Individuals with congenital or acquired deficiencies of the immune system are much more prone to serious infection. These 'experiments of nature' have shed considerable light on the functional significance of the deficient components.

It used to be thought that clinical immunodeficiency was confined to a few rare and rapidly fatal disorders but some forms are quite common, e.g. deficiencies of IgA or C2. Every practitioner should be aware of the major kinds of deficiency and ways in which they are diagnosed and managed. In the past they have often been missed and mismanaged.

Important clues

A diagnosis of immunodeficiency should always be considered when an individual experiences infection unusually frequently, in unusual locations or with unusual organisms and it should always form part of the differential diagnosis in children who 'fail to thrive'. The organisms involved may be unremarkable but infections with opportunistic organisms, i.e. those that do not usually cause disease, e.g. *Candida* or *Pneumocystis*, should arouse suspicion that immunity is defective. An increased susceptibility to infection can, however, be due to various non-immunological abnormalities which are considered briefly at the end of this chapter. Figure 13.1 indicates the major sites of involvement of the immune system in the immunodeficiency disorders which are reviewed in this chapter.

IMMUNODEFICIENCY DISORDERS

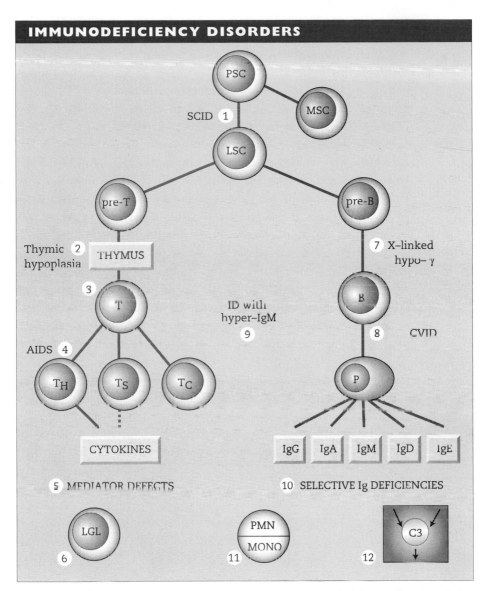

Fig. 13.1 Major sites of involvement in **immunodeficiency disorders** (ID)
(1) Severe combined immunodeficiency; (2) thymic hypoplasia; (3) T cell
deficiencies; (4) acquired immunodeficiency syndrome; (5) mediator
defects; (6) LGL defects; (7) X-linked hypogammaglobulinaemia;
(8) CVID (common variable immunodeficiency); (9) ID with hyper-IgM;
(10) selective immunoglobulin deficiencies, (11) phagocyte defects and
(12) complement deficiencies. PSC, pluripotent stem cell; MSC, myeloid
stem cell; LSC, lymphoid stem cell.

Investigation of suspected immunodeficiency

It is often difficult to decide when some children are experiencing more than their fair share of infection, particularly of the upper and lower respiratory tracts. The pattern of infection experienced by the patient often provides a useful clue to the nature of the underlying disorder (Table 13.1) and can simplify the process of investigation.

Initially, investigation should include a haemoglobin level, total and differential white cell count, platelet count, serum IgG, IgA, IgM, C3 and total haemolytic complement. A Schick test (to determine the anti-diphtheria response following previous immunization) and measurement of isohaemagglutinins may also be of value. If these investigations are normal and a high index of suspicion remains, or if specific pointers are already identified, then more detailed investigation is indicated. This may include characterization of T and B lymphocyte subpopulations, IgG subclasses, secretory IgA in saliva, more detailed complement assays and phagocyte function studies. *In vivo* challenge with pneumococcal vaccine, tetanus toxoid or dinitrochlorobenzene may be useful in assessing the severity of a particular defect.

PATTERNS OF INFECTION

Deficiency	Example	Pattern of infection
Stem cell	SCID	Viruses, fungi and bacteria
T cell	DiGeorge	Budding viruses, *Candida*, *Pneumocystis*
B cell	Hypogammaglobulinaemia	Pyogenic bacteria
Spleen	Splenectomy	Pneumococci, meningococci and H. influenzae
Phagocyte	CGD	Catalase-positive organisms e.g. staphylococci and *E. coli*
Phagocyte	LAD	Indolent infection with pyogenic bacteria; poor wound healing
Complement	C3	Pyogenic bacteria
Complement	C5, 6, 7, 8 or 9	*Neisseria* e.g. gonococci and meningococci

SCID, severe combined immunodeficiency; CGD, chronic granulomatous disease; LAD, leucocyte adhesion deficiency.

Table 13.1 Patterns of infection in selected immunodeficiency disorders.

Stem cell deficiency

This is the most severe defect of all and gives rise to **severe combined immunodeficiency** (SCID). It presents during the first few months of life with failure to thrive, persistent oral *Candida* infection, intractable diarrhoea and *Pneumocystis carinii* pneumonia. Infants often show a measles-like rash which may be due to a mild form of graft-versus-host disease following the transplacental passage of maternal lymphocytes. Maternal T cells have been identified in the circulation in some cases. Some patients lack other formed elements of the blood, e.g. polymorphonuclear leucocytes, because they have a defect which affects the myeloid stem cell as well (Fig. 13.1), a condition known as **reticular dysgenesis**. SCID infants may develop overwhelming infections with herpes and measles viruses, and inoculation with live vaccines, e.g. BCG or smallpox, is invariably fatal. Immunoglobulin levels are low and a proportion of cases have a homozygous deficiency of **adenosine deaminase** (ADA), which metabolizes adenosine and deoxyadenosine. Heterozygote carriers for this deficiency can be identified and antenatal diagnosis of the homozygous deficiency is possible. Rare individuals with a SCID-like syndrome fail to express HLA glycoproteins on the surface of their lymphocytes — a condition known as the **bare lymphocyte syndrome**.

Patients with SCID succumb during the first few years of life unless their stem cell deficiency is rectified by bone marrow transplantation. This requires the identification of a suitable donor, accurate HLA matching of donor and recipient, and graft acceptance by the latter. A further problem is the frequent development of **graft-versus-host (GVH) disease**, the incidence and severity of which can now be reduced by 'laundering' the graft to remove T cells using monoclonal antibodies or lectin columns (see Chapter 18). The use of fetal liver, fetal thymus or cultured thymic epithelium as sources of stem cells has been less successful. GVH can follow the transfusion of a single unit of stored blood and the T cells contained therein require elimination by irradiation before a blood transfusion is given to any patient who has defective cell-mediated immunity.

Thymic hypoplasia

The thymus, parathyroid glands, and parts of the face, jaw and great blood vessels, develop from the third and fourth pharyngeal arches between the sixth and eighth weeks of fetal life. In the **DiGeorge syndrome** their development is arrested, with the result that affected individuals lack a thymus (or have a few small fragments elsewhere in the neck), have hypoplastic parathyroid glands and abnormalities of their great vessels, e.g. transposition or Fallot's tetralogy, and may show facial abnormalities, e.g. low-set ears, small jaw and a short philtrum.

Medical attention is often sought because of congenital heart disease or hypocalcaemia due to parathormone deficiency but the triad of *Candida* infection, *Pneumocystis* pneumonia and persistent diarrhoea is soon evident. The absence of a thymic shadow on chest X-ray can be a useful pointer if thymic involution has not already occurred due to age or illness. The severity of the T cell defect is variable: most cases have a few T cells detectable in blood, and B cells and immunoglobulin levels are often normal. These individuals are less prone to develop GVH following blood transfusion and this is in keeping with their incomplete T cell defect. The immunological abnormality can be corrected by grafts of fetal thymus or the administration of thymic humoral factors. Partial forms of the DiGeorge syndrome are not uncommon and, if the cardiovascular abnormalities permit and the hypocalcaemia can be controlled by the administration of vitamin D and calcium supplements, the infants usually show a progressive increase in T cell numbers and function with age.

T cell deficiencies

Various T cell defects have been described without evidence of a primary thymic abnormality. Five are referred to here (Table 13.2), in addition to the acquired immunodeficiency syndrome (AIDS) (described in Chapter 12). T cell function can become abnormal for many other reasons, e.g. zinc deficiency (see Table 13.9), when lymphocytotoxins are present (as in various autoimmune diseases), and in many forms of secondary immunodeficiency (see p. 193 and Table 13.8).

T CELL DEFICIENCIES

Thymic hypoplasia (DiGeorge)
Purine nucleoside phosphorylase deficiency
Cartilage–hair hypoplasia
Wiskott–Aldrich syndrome
Ataxia telangiectasia
Chronic mucocutaneous candidiasis
Acquired immunodeficiency syndrome (AIDS)
  (see Chapter 12)

Table 13.2 T cell deficiencies.

PURINE NUCLEOSIDE PHOSPHORYLASE (PNP) DEFICIENCY

This, like the DiGeorge syndrome, is characterized by low T cell numbers with normal B cells and immunoglobulins but, in contrast, shows progressive deterioration rather than gradual improvement in immune status. These children are particularly susceptible to opportunistic viral infection and live vaccines can prove fatal. PNP is involved in the same purine salvage pathway as ADA and its deficiency is inherited as an autosomal recessive.

CARTILAGE–HAIR HYPOPLASIA

Some individuals present with abnormal T cell function, sparse thin hair, increased joint mobility and a form of short-limbed dwarfism. They are particularly prone to varicella infection, malabsorption and, in some instances, recurrent bacterial infection due to an associated neutropenia.

WISKOTT–ALDRICH SYNDROME

This X-linked disorder consists of severe eczema, thrombocytopenia and susceptibility to opportunistic infection and usually manifests itself during the first few months of life. Most children succumb to infection although intracranial haemorrhage and lymphomas also occur. Affected individuals show a progressive decline in T cell function with profound lymphopenia developing by the age of 6 years. The serum shows decreased IgM, increased IgA and IgE and normal IgG levels and an absence of antibodies reactive with polysaccharide antigens including blood group isohaemagglutinins. IgG or IgM monoclonal proteins are occasionally present. All the features of this syndrome can be corrected by bone marrow transplantation. In the absence of an available matched donor, splenectomy is useful in reducing the risk of bleeding. The underlying defect consists of the abnormal degradation of the major sialoglycoprotein (CD43) from the surface membrane of T cells and platelets. The defective gene has recently been located on the X chromosome but the protein it codes for has yet to be identified although it is known to be rich in proline residues.

ATAXIA TELANGIECTASIA

Cerebellar ataxia is first observed when affected children start to walk in their second year of life, although the dilated small blood vessels (telangiectasia) do not usually become apparent until several years later. Repeated respiratory tract infection is usually complicated by bronchiectasis but lymphoma (often of T cell origin) is a common cause of death. T cells (and particularly helper T cells) are reduced in number and function whereas B cells are normal or increased. IgA is low or absent, IgE is reduced, IgG levels are usually normal and IgM levels are often raised. Autoantibodies to IgA are often present. The condition is due to a DNA repair defect with increased susceptibility to form chromosomal breaks and translocations and is inherited as an autosomal recessive. Elevated levels of serum α-1-fetoprotein and carcino-embryonic antigen are also related to abnormal gene control. No satisfactory treatment is yet available for this progressive disorder. The effect of irradiation damage on peripheral blood lymphocytes can be used as a diagnostic test and chromosomal radiosensitivity may permit the detection of carriers.

CHRONIC MUCOCUTANEOUS CANDIDIASIS (CMCC)

This is a heterogeneous group of disorders characterized by chronic infection of skin, mouth and nails with *Candida*. Most patients have normal serum immunoglobulins and very high levels of anti-*Candida* antibody. It is classified into four immunological subsets:

Type I with normal *in vitro* T cell proliferation but impaired macrophage migration inhibition factor (MIF) production.

Type II with impaired lymphocyte proliferation and normal MIF production.

Type III showing impairment of both lymphocyte proliferation and MIF production.

Type IV in which no immunological abnormality is detected apart from the presence of a *Candida*-specific inhibitory factor present in serum.

Most CMCC patients with normal specific immune responses to *Candida* respond to the administration of iron and folate and it is likely that iron deficiency is a key factor in the development of chronic candidiasis in many of these individuals. Some have associated endocrine abnormalities, e.g. hypoparathyroidism, adrenal insufficiency and hypothyroidism.

Mediator defects

Lymphocytes produce a variety of soluble mediators or cytokines and the chemical characterization of some of them, e.g. interleukins and interferon, is well advanced (see Chapter 5). Impaired production of interleukin-2 is likely to be found whenever there is significant T cell deficiency but primary deficiencies of interleukins have yet to be described. Several reports point to the existence of patients who fail to produce interferon in response to viral infection and who are prone to develop fulminant hepatitis, herpes encephalitis or persistent Epstein–Barr virus infection. Defects of interferon production often go hand in hand with impaired natural killer (NK) cell activity and, in some instances, treatment with interferon has been shown to reverse an NK defect. Some children experiencing recurrent respiratory tract infection with rhinoviruses have deficient interferon responses and lack interferon in their nasal secretions. Deficient interferon production in leukaemia, systemic lupus and multiple sclerosis is likely to be a secondary phenomenon. Abnormalities of other cytokines have been described, e.g. impaired production of MIF in recurrent herpes simplex infection (cold sores) and in some patients with CMCC, but it is difficult to tell whether these abnormalities are primary or secondary.

Natural killer cell defects

Natural killer cells, alias large granular lymphocytes (LGL), are particularly effective at lysing virus-infected cells, some tumour cells and cells of bone marrow origin (see Chapter 10) and are activated by all three varieties of interferon and by interleukin-2. Interferon deficiency can be associated with NK deficiency and restoration of the former can correct the latter.

Patients with the **Chediak–Higashi syndrome** are prone to bacterial infection and the development of lymphomas, and their cells show absent NK activity although the oxidative burst is preserved. Their leucocytes and platelets contain abnormally large and misshapen lysosomal granules and it is likely that the granule abnormality is directly linked to their NK deficiency. A similar condition has been described in mutant Beige mice. Impaired NK activity occurs in a subset of patients with late-onset hypogammaglobulinaemia in association with a high incidence of autoimmune disease. NK abnormalities have also been reported in fatal infectious mononucleosis and malignant lymphoproliferative disease and it seems likely that this deficiency impairs defences against Epstein–Barr virus and so permits the inactivation or transformation of B lymphocytes.

B cell deficiencies—hypogammaglobulinaemia

An increased incidence of infection with pyogenic bacteria occurs with defects of antibody production or complement activation. This is because pus cells, i.e. neutrophil polymorphs, are the chief line of defence against these organisms and are recruited and activated following the interaction

TYPES OF HYPOGAMMAGLOBULINAEMIA

Primary	Secondary
Bruton's disease (X-LA)	Myelomatosis
Immunodeficiency with hyper-IgM	Chronic lymphatic leukaemia
Common variable immunodeficiency	Protein-losing enteropathy
Selective immunoglobulin deficiencies	Congenital rubella
With thymoma	
With dwarfism	
Transcobalamin II deficiency	
Transient hypogammaglobulinaemia of infancy	

Table 13.3 Examples of primary and secondary hypogammaglobulinaemia.

of specific antibody and complement. The major varieties of generalized antibody deficiency are described in this section (Table 13.3). Complement deficiencies are described on p. 191–192.

X-LINKED HYPOGAMMAGLOBULINAEMIA

Bruton's disease (X-LA)

The classical form of antibody deficiency was described by Bruton in 1952 and is usually referred to as **X-linked agammaglobulinaemia (or X-LA)** as there is a complete absence of γ globulin. Affected males usually present with recurrent infection at between 4 months and 2 years of age and are protected from earlier infection because of the placental transfer of maternal IgG antibody. *Haemophilus influenzae*, *Streptococcus pneumoniae* and staphylococci are the most frequent causes and the respiratory tract and skin the most frequent sites of infection. Episodes of diarrhoea may occur and are often due to infection with *Giardia lamblia*. A minority of patients develop arthritis which can be due to mycoplasma and responds to immunoglobulin replacement and chemotherapy. A few patients develop encephalitis (sometimes in association with dermatomyositis) due to an echovirus and although this can respond to vigorous immunoglobulin replacement it is often progressive. Other virus infections are not usually a problem although paralytic poliomyelitis can follow immunization with the live attenuated vaccine.

The defect is one of inability of pre-B cells to differentiate into B cells (Fig. 13.1) and this has recently been shown to be due to the lack of a **B cell-specific tyrosine kinase** which has a critical role in B cell development. Very few B cells or plasma cells are found in affected individuals whereas pre-B cells are present in normal numbers in bone marrow and show the typical absence of surface immunoglobulin in conjunction with the presence of cytoplasmic μ heavy chains. IgM and IgA are usually absent in serum and secretions and serum IgG levels are low but rarely completely absent. T cell numbers and function are usually normal. Male infants at risk should have their circulating B cell levels measured rather than wait for maternal antibody to decay so that replacement therapy can be started promptly.

A combination of immunoglobulin replacement therapy, rigorous use of antibacterial agents, and measures designed to achieve maximal drainage of infected sites form the basis of the long-term management of generalized antibody deficiencies of all kinds. Immunoglobulin replacement was traditionally administered by intramuscular injection at weekly intervals but preparations are now available for intravenous and subcutaneous use. The latter not only require less frequent administration but can be given by the patients themselves, after appropriate tuition. The initiation of immunoglobulin replacement therapy can be as dramatically beneficial as the introduction of insulin therapy to the type I diabetic and, in both situations, careful follow-up is required for life.

Immunodeficiency with hyper-IgM

This X-linked condition is characterized by a profound lack of IgG and IgA but an increased level of polyclonal IgM (which distinguishes it from macroglobulinaemia which is described on p. 250). These patients are prone to pyogenic infections and may also develop neutropenia and thrombocytopenia due to the presence of IgM autoantibodies to neutrophils and platelets. They show lymphoid hyperplasia (but lack germinal centres) and have an increased incidence of lymphoma. Serum IgM levels and the associated lymphoid hyperplasia may decline when immunoglobulin replacement is given.

The underlying defect has recently been identified as the lack of a glycoprotein (gp39) normally expressed on the surface of activated T cells with which the B cell CD40 membrane protein interacts during the formation of memory B cells; enabling the switch from IgM to other isotypes characteristic of the response to T-dependent antigens.

COMMON VARIABLE IMMUNODEFICIENCY (CVID)

This is more common and less consistent than the X-linked forms. It usually presents well after infancy and most often in the third decade and has also been referred to as late-onset hypogammaglobulinaemia. The pattern of infection is, however, similar and chiefly affects the lungs, sinuses and gastrointestinal tract. Herpes zoster infection, meningitis, osteomyelitis and skin sepsis also occur. Some patients develop malabsorption due to bowel infection with *Giardia*, *Campylobacter* or *Cryptosporidium*. Gastric atrophy and achlorhydria occur in about a third of patients and often associate with vitamin B_{12} deficiency although the typical autoantibodies are not detectable and a diagnosis of classical pernicious anaemia is debatable. There is also an increased incidence of gastric carcinoma.

Nodular lymphoid hyperplasia is often found in the gut. The nodules occur in the small bowel, resemble Peyer's patches and consist mostly of B lymphocytes. They are usually seen in patients with circulating B lymphocytes and preserved IgM production. Sarcoid-like granulomata are another feature of CVID and are found in the lungs, liver, spleen and skin although no associated microorganisms have been identified. Hepatosplenomegaly is the main clinical feature and can be controlled with steroid therapy. Autoimmune haemolytic anaemia, thrombocytopenia and neutropenia are other complications seen in this group; these usually respond to steroids or may require a cytotoxic agent, e.g. vincristine.

CVID is often familial but there is no clear pattern of inheritance. Although the exact nature of the immunological defect is uncertain, cases divide into three main groups in which B cells fail to differentiate into plasma cells (Fig. 13.1):

1 those with an intrinsic B cell defect;
2 those with an immunoregulatory T cell imbalance; and
3 those with autoantibodies to T or B lymphocytes.

In the first instance the B lymphocytes appear to be immature. In the second instance B lymphocytes are probably normal but fail to differentiate due to either a lack of helper T cells or overactivity of a suppressor T population. Some patients with late-onset disease have low NK activity.

Treatment is as for the X-linked deficiency, i.e. immunoglobulin replacement, antibacterial agents and drainage of infected sites with careful follow-up concerning the other complications to which these patients are prone.

OTHER FORMS OF HYPOGAMMAGLOBULINAEMIA (Table 13.3)

Patients with a thymoma often have an immunological disorder. Myasthenia gravis is the most common, with red cell aplasia and hypogammaglobulinaemia occurring in 10–20 per cent of cases. These patients lack pre-B and B cells. Excessive activity of the suppressor T cell population may be responsible for inactivation of the B cell series. Removal of the tumour can reverse the red cell aplasia but has no effect on the antibody deficiency.

Various kinds of dwarfism associate with isolated B cell deficiency one of which is associated growth hormone deficiency. Hypogammaglobulinaemia also occurs in an inherited deficiency of transcobalamin II, which can be reversed by giving large doses of vitamin B_{12}.

Transient hypogammaglobulinaemia of infancy

This condition is probably underdiagnosed and occurs during the period when maternally derived IgG wanes and the infant's own antibodies appear (IgM followed by IgG and IgA). The trough of antibody level usually occurs between the third and sixth months of life but can be more prolonged and is usually more severe in premature infants. Affected infants often develop troublesome infection; they have normal B cells but a relative lack of T helper cells. Some have immunodeficient relatives. The antibody deficiency usually resolves by the age of 2 years and immunoglobulin replacement is required until normal levels are attained.

Severe antibody deficiency can occur as a secondary phenomenon in a number of other diseases, e.g. protein-losing enteropathy (classically seen in intestinal lymphangiectasia), myelomatosis, chronic lymphocytic leukaemia and congenital rubella. Immunoglobulin replacement can be of value in addition to measures directed toward the primary abnormality.

Selective immunoglobulin deficiencies

IgG DEFICIENCY

As IgG accounts for 67 per cent of serum IgG, a deficiency of this subclass will usually be diagnosed as CVID (and some of these patients lack IgA as well). The commonest IgG subclass abnormality in adults is deficiency of IgG_3 whereas in children it is IgG_2. Many normal individuals lack detectable levels of IgG_4. Antibodies reactive with the polysaccharide capsules of pyogenic bacteria such as pneumococci and *H. influenzae* are mostly of IgG_2 isotype. Serious infections are associated with IgG_2 deficiency even when the total serum IgG level is within the normal range. Recurrent bacterial infection also complicates IgG_3 deficiency but the mechanism is poorly understood. In either case, immunoglobulin replacement is effective in preventing infection.

IgA DEFICIENCY

IgA deficiency is the commonest form of immunodeficiency among Caucasians, occurring in about 1 in 600 of the population. Most cases are sporadic but some have family members with varied forms of antibody deficiency. It has been noted in patients treated with phenytoin or penicillamine, although the underlying susceptibility to develop IgA deficiency may be part of the primary disease for which they receive these treatments, i.e. epilepsy or rheumatoid arthritis. There is good evidence of an association between possession of the HLA A1, B8, DR3 haplotype and IgA deficiency. IgA deficiency is also a marked feature of ataxia telangiectasia (see p. 179). Patients lacking IgA are prone to sinopulmonary infection and bowel colonization with *Giardia*, *Salmonella* and other enteric pathogens. Sporadic reports have pointed to a higher incidence of viral hepatitis, type 1 diabetes and other autoimmune disorders, and this susceptibility is probably due to defective handling of enteroviruses. Atopic disorders (see p. 229) are also more common in IgA-deficient individuals.

Almost all IgA-deficient patients possess circulating B cells bearing surface IgA but these appear immature, often coexpress IgM and fail to differentiate into IgA-secreting plasma cells. In some cases plasma cells producing the IgA2 subclass are present in the gut with the defect confined to IgA1-producing bone marrow plasma cells; in others, both subclasses are deficient. Circulating T cells which block the differentiation of IgA plasma cells have been identified in some patients with IgA deficiency.

IgM DEFICIENCY

Selective deficiency of this isotype is rare. Such patients lack isohaemagglutinins and are particularly susceptible to meningitis and septicaemia with encapsulated organisms, e.g. pneumococci and meningococci.

IMMUNOGLOBULIN COMPONENT DEFICIENCIES

Kappa chain, lambda chain and secretory component deficiencies have each been described in association with increased susceptibility to infection. In the last case, neither IgA nor secretory component is detectable in saliva or jejunal fluid whereas the serum IgA level is normal. J chain deficiency has not yet been described but might be expected to give a selective abnormality with normal levels of monomeric IgG, IgA and IgM but absence of the polymeric forms of IgA and IgM.

Phagocyte defects

Phagocytes, i.e, neutrophil polymorphs and monocytes, have a critical role in defence against many bacterial pathogens. Profound neutropenia is associated with infection, septicaemia and ulceration of the mouth, skin and respiratory tract. Phagocyte function divides into three sequential components: (i) mobility, margination and adherence, (ii) phagocytosis, and (iii) intracellular killing (see Chapter 8). The primary phagocyte defects described below illustrate the importance of these different processes (Table 13.4). It is important to realize, however, that the presence of infection itself can cause secondary alterations in phagocyte performance. This may be due to toxic or inhibitory factors produced during infection or result from the recruitment of more mature cells, leaving earlier forms to predominate in the blood (often referred to as a 'left shift' in the segmentation pattern of neutrophil nuclei when viewing the blood film). In some families a cyclical neutropenia (with a periodicity of 3–4 weeks) can occur and serial studies may be required to identify this problem.

DEFECTS OF MOBILITY AND PHAGOCYTOSIS

Various abnormalities have been described which affect the ability of phagocytes to migrate to sites of infection. This process involves margination and adherence to endothelial membranes, a directed response to chemotactic stimuli, and adherence at the site of antibody combination and complement fixation. Immune adherence is intimately linked to phagocytosis and it is rare to find defects of phagocytosis alone. Not all mobility abnormalities are, however, associated with detectable abnormalities of phagocytosis.

PHAGOCYTE DEFECTS

Mobility ± phagocytosis	Killing
Leucocyte adhesion deficiency	· Chronic granulomatous disease
Schwachman's syndrome	· Myeloperoxidase deficiency
Absent specific granules	G6PD deficiency
Chediak–Higashi syndrome	

Table 13.4 Primary phagocyte defects.

Leucocyte adhesion deficiency

These patients usually present with infections of the skin, mouth, respiratory tract and around the rectum but with little evidence of pus formation. Abscesses tend to be 'cold' and their pus 'thin'. Periodontal disease is common. Wound healing is impaired and delayed separation of the umbilical cord is a feature of some cases.

This condition is characterized by a failure of neutrophils and monocytes to migrate to sites of tissue infection (in spite of persisting neutrophilia). It has recently become clear that although the clinical manifestations vary considerably between cases, this group of disorders is due to a defect in the biosynthesis of the β chain (CD18) common to three glycoproteins (of c. 150 000 kD) normally present on the surface of leucocytes. These three **integrin receptors** are known as LFA-1, p150/95 and CR3 (the iC3b receptor) and each possess a different α chain (Table 13.5). Neutrophils, monocytes and NK cells possess all three heterodimers whereas B and T lymphocytes only express LFA-1. Defective synthesis of the β component results in impaired or absent expression of αβ complexes on the cell surface. The condition is usually inherited as an autosomal recessive and several different mutations of the CD18 gene have been described. Patients with complete CD18 deficiency usually die in early life but those with partial defects benefit from prophylactic and acute administration of antibiotics. Bone marrow transplantation has been successful in correcting this condition.

Schwachman's syndrome, in which neutropenia associates with exocrine pancreatic insufficiency and growth retardation, is another example of a neutrophil mobility defect due to a defective membrane protein. Cells from patients with the **Chediak–Higashi syndrome** also show defective mobility but with normal phagocytosis. They contain giant secondary lysosomes which contain the products of fusion of many cytoplasmic granules and the functional abnormalities observed may well

INTEGRIN RECEPTORS			
Integrin receptor	α chain	β chain	Ligands
LFA-1	CD11a	CD18	ICAM 1 & 2
p150/95	CD11b	CD18	iC3b
CR3	CD11c	CD18	iC3b

Table 13.5 Integrin receptors and their ligands.

be a consequence of the continuous activation which these cells undergo. They fail to kill catalase-positive or catalase-negative organisms and have absent NK activity although the oxidative burst is preserved, suggesting that the granule abnormality is directly linked to the NK deficiency. Some patients with recurrent infection and impaired neutrophil mobility have a **congenital absence of specific granules** but it is not clear whether the abnormality is due to lactoferrin deficiency or a reduction in receptors for chemotactic factors.

Hyper-IgE syndrome

This disorder is characterized by a chronic eczematous dermatitis in association with recurrent skin, lung and bone abscesses, otitis media and sinusitis. The dermatitis and proneness to infection is usually evident within the first 6 weeks of life. Most infections are due to *Staphylococcus aureus* but candida infections are also common and may take the form of chronic mucocutaneous candidiasis (see p. 180). These patients often have coarse facial features, osteoporosis, and are prone to bone fractures. They have extremely high serum levels of total IgE (usually > 5000 IU ml⁻¹), raised levels of histamine in blood and urine, and eosinophilia. The condition can be familial but the pattern of inheritance is unclear. The frequent occurrence of skin abscesses, which show little surrounding erythema, gave rise to the earlier description of 'Job's syndrome' but the term **hyper-IgE (HIE) syndrome** is currently preferred. These patients possess normal numbers of neutrophils which phagocytose and kill normally but respond poorly to chemotactic stimuli. The raised levels of histamine may have a role in the inhibition of neutrophil chemotaxis which can be reversed by histamine (H_2) antagonists. However, it has also been shown that a chemotactic inhibitory factor of 61 000 kD is produced by mononuclear cells from patients with HIE syndrome, and activation of these cells may also lead to the bone demineralization observed in these patients.

Phagocyte mobility is secondarily impaired in various other disorders. The effect of infection has already been emphasized but impairment also occurs in malnutrition, burns, diabetes, uraemia and following the administration of various drugs and anaesthetic agents.

DEFECTS OF INTRACELLULAR KILLING

The archetype is the rare but much studied disorder **chronic granulomatous disease** (CGD). Phagocytosis is normal but oxidative killing is absent in both neutrophils and monocytes. It is usually X-linked and affected male children develop infection — often taking the form of abscesses — of lungs, lymph nodes, liver and bones. Wound healing is slow and sinus formation may follow attempts at drainage. Other features include splenomegaly and gastrointestinal involvement. The pattern of organ involvement is probably due to the uptake of neutrophils containing intracellular pathogens by fixed macrophages in bone marrow, liver, lungs and lymph nodes, where chronic granulomata develop and are difficult to eradicate.

The defect arises because of a failure to generate an effective membrane NADPH oxidase to initiate the oxidative burst which normally accompanies phagocytosis (see p. 118). CGD monocytes are also less efficient at antigen processing and presentation. The molecular cause of most cases of membrane oxidase deficiency is defective production of the heavy chain of the cytochrome b involved in the electron transport chain linked to the membrane oxidase. Most of the problem organisms for patients with CGD are **catalase-positive**, i.e. they destroy any excess hydrogen peroxide they produce. Examples include many staphylococci, *Escherichia coli*, *Serratia marcescens*, *Salmonella*, *Aspergillus*, *Candida* and atypical mycobacteria. In contrast, organisms which generate H_2O_2 and are catalase-negative, e.g. *H. influenzae* and streptococci, do not cause persistent infection. The reason for this disparity is that hydrogen peroxide produced in the absence of catalase can be incorporated into the metabolic pathway of the phagocyte to compensate for the lack of endogenous H_2O_2 production so that, in effect, the pathogen commits suicide (Table 13.6).

The outlook for what was previously known as 'fatal granulomatous disease of childhood' has improved with the use of cell-penetrating antibacterial agents, e.g. trimethoprim and rifampicin, and an increasing number of patients are now surviving into adulthood. More recently, treatment with recombinant human IFN-γ has been shown to enhance the respiratory burst and bactericidal activity and produce clinical improvement in some patients with CGD. This effect is thought to follow increased expression of the gene for the cytochrome b heavy chain.

Several other enzyme deficiencies have been proposed as causes of defective phagocyte killing, e.g. deficiencies of myeloperoxidase and glucose-6-phosphate dehydrogenase (G6PD). In the former case the enzyme is deficient in neutrophils and monocytes although eosinophil peroxidase is preserved. Deficiency of either enzyme gives a clinical picture resembling CGD although the individuals are less incapacitated.

Complement deficiencies

Heritable deficiencies of each of the nine components of the classical pathway (including the three subunits of C1) as well as properdin, factor D and the inhibitors of C1 (C1 esterase inhibitor) and C3 (H and I) have been identified in man. Major deficiencies of C3 are associated with severe bacterial infection; deficiencies of components of the membrane attack pathway give increased susceptibility to infection with *Neisseria*, e.g. gonococci and meningococci; whereas deficiencies of early components in the classical pathway are associated with various forms of immune complex disease rather than overt infection (Table 13.7). Deficiency of the C1 esterase inhibitor is the cause of **hereditary angio-oedema**. Deficiency of the alternative pathway component, properdin, is associated with severe bacterial infection, particularly with neisserial

CGD NEUTROPHILS AND AEROBIC ORGANISMS

Neutrophil	Microbe status		Result
	H_2O_2	Catalase	
Normal	+	+	Oxidative lysis
Normal	+	−	Oxidative lysis
CGD		+	Microbial persistence
CGD	+	−	Microbial suicide

CGD, chronic granulomatous disease.

Table 13.6 Outcome of interaction between normal or CGD neutrophils and aerobic organisms.

COMPLEMENT DEFICIENCIES

Component	Clinical picture
C1 esterase inhibitor	Hereditary angio-oedema Immune complex disease
C1q, C1r, C1s C4 C2	Immune complex disease e.g. systemic lupus, vasculitis and glomerulonephritis
C3, factor I, factor H	Pyogenic infection
C5, C6, C7, C8, C9 Properdin, factor D	Gonococcal and meningococcal infection

Table 13.7 Clinical associations of primary complement deficiencies.

organisms. Factor D deficiency also associates with neisserial infection but is more benign. A relatively common defect (5 per cent of the Caucasoid population) of complement-mediated opsonization has recently been shown to be due to deficiency of **mannose-binding protein** (MBP). This protein binds to mannose and N-acetylglucosamine on microbial cell walls and activates C3 by a C1q-independent route. MBP deficiency not only gives rise to pyogenic infections in infancy, chronic diarrhoea and failure to thrive but adults who are homozygous for abnormalities of this protein are also prone to recurrent infection.

Each of the deficiencies listed is inherited in autosomal recessive mode except for properdin deficiency, which is X-linked, and hereditary angio-oedema, which occurs as an autosomal dominant. C2 deficiency is the most common: approximately 1 per cent of the population are heterozygous for the deficient gene which occurs in linkage disequilibrium with HLA DR2 (see p. 236).

The cleavage products of C3 have a pre-eminent role in defence against pyogenic bacteria and the fact that only major deficiencies of C3 associate with severe infection emphasizes the importance of the alternative pathway in achieving C3 conversion when classical pathway components are deficient (see Chapter 7). Components of the membrane attack pathway only seem to be indispensable with regard to neisserial infections. The association of defects in the classical pathway with **immune complex disease** is a consequence of the role of these components in inhibiting the precipitation of immune complexes and facilitating their clearance from the circulation (see pp. 107 & 232). Deficiency of either of the two C3 control proteins (factor H – C3b binding protein – and factor I – the C3b inactivator) permits the unchecked activation of C3, leading to secondary C3 deficiency with a pattern of infection very similar to that found in primary C3 deficiency.

HEREDITARY ANGIO-OEDEMA (HAO)

This condition usually presents by the age of 10 with episodes of subepithelial oedema of the skin, larynx or gastrointestinal tract which last for 2–3 days. Oedema of the gut can present as severe abdominal pain and laryngeal oedema can prove fatal. C1 esterase inhibitor inactivates various serine esterases including plasmin, kallikrein, and activated factor XI and factor XII (Hageman factor) as well as the activated forms of C1 (C$\overline{1}$r and C$\overline{1}$s). In its absence, C1 becomes readily cleaved (especially at extravascular sites where levels of another major enzyme inhibitor – α_2-macroglobulin – are very low) with generation of the activated forms of C4 and C2 and, in particular, a vasoactive peptide derived from C2b by plasmin. This process does not cause effective C3 conversion as it mostly occurs in fluid phase without the generation of a stable membrane-bound C3 convertase (see Chapter 7). Thus these patients have low levels of C4 and C2 with normal C3.

The large majority of patients are heterozygous for C1 esterase inhibitor deficiency but their inhibitor levels are usually well below 50 per cent normal because of increased catabolism. A rarer form consists of heterozygosity for a dysfunctional form of the inhibitor. Patients with HAO also have an increased susceptibility to immune complex disease probably as a consequence of their secondary deficiencies of C2 and C4. The condition can be treated by giving inhibitors of fibrinolysis, e.g. ε-amino caproic acid and tranexamic acid, or the administration of androgenic steroids, e.g. danazol or stanozolol. The latter increase synthesis of the inhibitor and correct the C2 and C4 deficiency. Purified C1 esterase inhibitor is now available for replacement therapy by intravenous injection.

Acquired forms of C1 esterase inhibitor are usually associated with lymphoproliferative disease. This has been variously attributed to absorption of the inhibitor protein by tumour cells, the formation of anti-idiotype complexes or the presence of a monoclonal autoantibody which inactivates the inhibitor.

Secondary forms of immunodeficiency

The commonest cause of serious immunodeficiency in clinical practice is none of the above but rather the impact that a number of diseases and the therapies used to treat them have upon the immune system. Table 13.8 lists some of the more important examples. Depression of T cell responses occurs early on in Hodgkin's disease whereas antibody deficiency is usually a progressive feature of chronic lymphocytic leukaemia and myeloma. Other disorders associated with impaired protein intake or protein loss also cause immunodeficiency and secondary impairment develops during the course of most forms of chronic inflammatory disease.

LYMPHOID ABLATION

The surgical removal of tonsils, adenoids, appendix or local lymph nodes has little effect on immunological responsiveness although one should be reluctant to remove lymphoid tissue in individuals who already show signs of immunodeficiency. Removal of the spleen, however, greatly increases the risk of fulminant infection with pneumococci, meningococci

CAUSES OF SECONDARY IMMUNODEFICIENCY

Leukaemia, e.g. chronic lymphatic leukaemia
Lymphoma, e.g. Hodgkin's disease
Myeloma
Malnutrition
Burns
Nephrotic syndrome
Protein-losing enteropathy
Uraemia
Down's syndrome
Chronic inflammatory disease
Persistent infection, e.g. malaria or leprosy
Congenital viral infection, e.g. rubella
Immunosuppressive drugs
Ablation of lymphoid tissue by surgery or
    irradiation

Table 13.8 Major causes of secondary immunodeficiency.

and *H. influenzae*. The risk is greatest in the first few years of life and within 5 years of splenectomy. Polyvalent pneumococcal vaccine should be given (and, where possible, before splenectomy is performed) in conjunction with prophylactic antibiotics. The immunological changes consist of impaired clearance of intravascular organisms, reduced concentrations of serum complement and IgM, and a disturbance of the normal profile of lymphocyte subpopulations, often with a moderate lymphocytosis.

Whole body irradiation with X-rays has powerful immunosuppressive effects, especially on the T cell compartment, and the technique of total lymphoid irradiation developed for the treatment of Hodgkin's disease has a profound and selective effect on T cell function. It has been used to facilitate graft acceptance and for the treatment of refractory autoimmune disease and appears to act as much by inducing suppression as by ablating help.

The use of powerful immunosuppressive drugs, e.g. corticosteroids, cytotoxic agents and antilymphocyte globulin, can also cause profound impairment of the immune system. The suppression of graft rejection in transplant recipients is still a balancing act between the development of serious infective complications due to generalized immunosuppression (particularly of T cell responses), on the one hand, and loss of the graft due to T cell-mediated rejection, on the other. The pattern of infection seen in these individuals is reminiscent of the problems experienced by individuals with primary T cell defects (see Table 13.1).

Non-immunological abnormalities which predispose to infection (see Table 13.9)

The skin and other epithelial surfaces of the body provide an important first line of defence against infection. Denuded areas of skin, e.g. in severe **eczema** or following **burns**, provide ready access for many organisms. Lysozyme is a bacteriostatic component of mucous secretions, and the acid pH of the skin, gastric juice and vaginal secretions normally inhibit the growth of many microorganisms. Hidradenitis suppurativa is a dominantly inherited disorder in which an abnormality of the apocrine glands causes obstruction of their ducts resulting in infection in the axillary and inguinal regions and around the umbilicus and areola of the breast.

Kartagener's syndrome is a form of ciliary dyskinesia in which an intrinsic defect in ciliary function (absence of the ATPase containing dynein arms) causes defective mucociliary clearance and pulmonary, nasal and middle ear disease, and impaired sperm motility. In **cystic fibrosis**, ciliary function is normal but impaired clearance is due to abnormalities of the mucus component. Impaired drainage of any duct or hollow viscus provokes infection whether it is due to congenital malformation or the damaging effects of infection itself, e.g. bronchiectasis.

NON-IMMUNOLOGICAL ABNORMALITIES

Affected site	Disorder
Skin	Burns and trauma
	Eczema
	Hidradenitis suppurativa
Mucosa	Ciliary dyskinesia
	Cystic fibrosis
Impaired drainage of a duct or hollow viscus	e.g. Bronchiectasis
Cofactor deficiencies	
Zinc	Acrodermatitis enteropathica
Iron	Mucocutaneous candidiasis (see p. 180)
Acid pH	Vaginal candidiasis
Cortisol	Addison's disease
Insulin	Diabetes mellitus
Vitamin B_{12}	Transcobalamin deficiency

Table 13.9 Examples of non-immunological abnormalities associated with susceptibility to infection.

Infection can follow alteration in the level of various other cofactors, e.g. zinc, iron and iron-binding proteins, vitamin B_{12}, cortisol, insulin and interferon. The free iron level may be especially critical. The over-energetic treatment of the anaemia of infection with iron supplementation can exacerbate infection (many bacteria utilize iron), yet some patients with chronic candidiasis respond favourably to iron treatment. The levels of acute phase proteins (e.g. C-reactive protein) adapt to infective stimuli (via interleukin release) but deficiency of acute phase proteins with antienzyme activity can cause tissue destruction without overt infection, e.g. α_1-antitrypsin deficiency and pulmonary emphysema.

KEY POINTS

1 Imunodeficiency should be suspected when an individual experiences infections occurring unusually frequently, in unusual locations or with unusual organisms.
2 The pattern of infection often points to the nature of the defect which may be located in almost any part of the immune system.
3 Severe combined immunodeficiency (SCID) and T cell defects often present in the first few weeks of life whereas B cell defects do not become apparent for at least 3 months (when the level of maternal immunoglobulin has waned) and sometimes present many years later.
4 The defective genes have been identified in several immunodeficiency disorders, e.g. SCID, Bruton's hypogammaglobulinaemia, immunodeficiency with hyper-IgM, and chronic granulomatous disease.
5 The commonest forms of immunodeficiency are secondary to other diseases or are a side-effect of therapy, e.g. with immunosuppressive drugs.
6 The prompt diagnosis and treatment of immunodeficiency disorders can have a major and life-long impact on the affected individual.

Further reading

Arnaout M.A. & Newburger P.E. (1993) Leucocyte adhesion molecule deficiency and chronic granulomatous disease. In Lachmann P.J., Peters D.K., Rosen F.S. & Walport M.J. eds, *Clinical Aspects of Immunology*, 5th edn. Blackwell Scientific Publications, Oxford.

Chapel H.M. for the Consensus Panel. (1994) Consensus on diagnosis and management of primary antibody deficiencies. *British Medical Journal*, **308**, 581–585.

Jefferis R. & Kumararatne D.S. (1990) Selective IgG subclass deficiency: quantification and clinical relevance. *Clinical and Experimental Immunology*, **81**, 357–367.

Lachmann P.J. (1993) Complement deficiencies – genetic and acquired. In Lachmann P.J., Peters D.K., Rosen F.S. & Walport M.J. eds, *Clinical Aspects of Immunology*, 5th edn. Blackwell Scientific Publications, Oxford.

Ochs H.D. & Aruffo A. (1993) Advances in X-linked immunodeficiency diseases. *Current*

Opinion in Pediatrics, **5**, 684–691.

Rosen F.S. & Seligmann M. eds (1993) *Immunodeficiencies*. Harwood, Philadelphia.

Rosen F.S., Cooper M.D. & Wedgwood R.J.P. (1995) The primary immunodeficiencies. *New England Journal of Medicine*, **333**, 431–440.

Summerfield J.A., Ryder S, Sumiya M. et al. (1995) Mannose-binding protein gene mutations associated with unusual and severe infections in adults. *Lancet*, **345**, 886–889.

CHAPTER 14

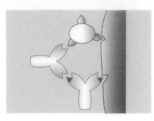

Allergy and
Autoimmunity

The primary role of the immune system is to protect the host against infection with pathogenic organisms. However, the enormity and intricacy of this task (discussed in Chapter 11) means that survival is often achieved 'at a price' which usually involves appreciable inflammatory damage to host tissues during the course of infection. In addition, the immune response is prone to be activated by extrinsic antigens of a non-microbial nature, and during the course of other diseases it may focus its attention on components of self, i.e. autoantigens. In some otherwise well-documented immunologically mediated diseases the definitive antigens have yet to be identified. This chapter reviews these four categories of immunological disease which together constitute a major part of **immunopathology**.

Responses to microbial antigens

Inflammation is a well-known consequence of infection and its classical signs of **rubor** (erythema), **tumor** (swelling), **calor** (heat) and **dolor** (pain) were described by Celsus c. AD 30. However, the subsequent identification of noxious materials produced by pathogens, e.g. diphtheria and cholera toxins, led to the general view that much of the pathology of infectious disease was due to the evils of the infecting organism whose ill effects the immune response was endeavouring to contain. It is now clear that much of the discomfort and disability is often a direct consequence of the activities of the immune response against the pathogen and this is well illustrated by studies performed with lymphocytic choriomeningitis (LCM) virus.

If adult mice of a certain strain are inoculated with LCM virus they develop fits and paralysis due to an acute encephalitis (Fig. 14.1). If

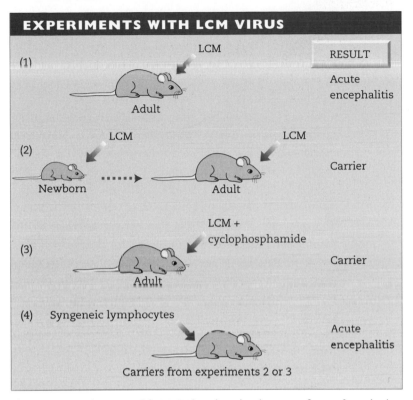

Fig. 14.1 Experiments with LCM virus in mice (see text for explanation)

Inoculation is performed when the animals are newborn they do not become ill, even when reinoculated as adults, although they remain lifelong carriers of the virus. If adult animals are given a single dose of a cytotoxic drug—cyclophosphamide—shortly after the inoculation of LCM virus they too suffer no ill effects and continue to harbour the virus. Either of these two 'carrier states' can be rapidly terminated by the administration of histocompatible lymphocytes from a normal animal (experiment 4, Fig. 14.1). These findings indicate that the carrier animals lack lymphocytes capable of responding to LCM; the severity of the tissue damage being governed by the vigour of the immune response rather than the continued presence of the virus. Specific responsiveness can be subverted by administering the virus before the animal is immunologically mature or eliminated by the administration of a drug which kills the specifically reactive cells of the immune response as they proliferate in response to the introduction of the virus.

There are many examples of infections in which there is good evidence for a major contribution by the immune response to the tissue damage which ensues, and some of these are listed in Table 14.1. Massive inflammatory lung damage occurs in acute bacterial **pneumonia** and, even today, this condition carries a mortality rate of about 10 per cent even when appropriate antibacterial agents are used. Several of the important organisms concerned, e.g. pneumococci, staphylococci and *Legionella*, possess subtle ways of evading the immune response (see Chapter 11). Much of the tissue destruction (caseation) seen in postprimary **pulmonary tuberculosis** is due to the intensity of the cell-mediated immune response to the *Mycobacterium*: the latter presents particular problems to the immune response because of its waxy coat and intracellular location. Infection with *Mycobacterium leprae* is also very difficult for the immune response to eradicate and individuals may show dramatic signs of tissue destruction (tuberculoid leprosy) or the immune response may become overwhelmed (lepromatous leprosy). Most of the tissue damage seen in secondary and tertiary **syphilis** is immunologically mediated. The severity of infective serum **hepatitis** is largely determined by the intensity of the immune response, and acute infection of the throat with certain strains of β-haemolytic streptococci can be followed by inflammation of the heart and joints (**rheumatic fever**), basal ganglia (**chorea**, i.e. involuntary movements) and kidneys (**glomerulonephritis**).

Table 14.2 includes a list of several organ-based diseases associated with immune responses to microbial antigens. The skin is a frequent battle-ground for immune responses and **leprosy** and **erythema nodosum** are just two examples: the latter is characterized by tender red nodules which often follow streptococcal infection. **Scleritis** produces a painful red eye, can lead to blindness, and may follow infection

TISSUE DAMAGE IN INFECTION

Disease	Infectious agent
Acute pneumonia	*Pneumococcus*
	Staphylococcus
	Legionella
Pulmonary tuberculosis	*Mycobacterium tuberculosis*
Tuberculoid leprosy	*M. leprae*
Syphilis	*Treponema pallidum*
Serum hepatitis	*Hepatitis B virus*
Glomerulonephritis	*Streptococcus*
	Plasmodium malariae
Rheumatic fever	*Streptococcus*

Table 14.1 Some infectious diseases or their complications in which immunologically mediated tissue damage is a major feature.

ANTIGEN-TRIGGERED DISEASES

	1. Microbial antigens	2. Non-microbial antigens	3. Autoantigens	4. Unidentified antigens

Skin	Leprosy
	Erythema
	  nodosum
		Atopic dermatitis
		Dermatitis
		  herpetiformis
			Pemphigus
			Pemphigoid
				Cutaneous
				  vasculitis

Eyes/nose	Scleritis
	Reiter's
	  syndrome
		Allergic
		  conjunctivitis
		Allergic rhinitis
			Lens-induced uveitis
			Keratoconjunctivitis
			  sicca
				Other forms of
				  uveitis
				Nasal polyposis

Lungs	Bacterial
	  pneumonia
	Pulmonary
	  tuberculosis
		Allergic asthma
		Allergic alveolitis
			Anti-glomerular
			  basement
			  membrane
			  (GBM) disease
				Pulmonary
				  eosinophilia
				Sarcoidosis

Gut	Enteric fever Chronic gastritis	Food allergy Coeliac disease	Pernicious anaemia	Crohn's disease Ulcerative colitis

Kidneys	Poststreptococcal
	  nephritis
	Malarial nephritis
		Seasonal nephrotic
		  syndrome
			Anti-GBM disease
			Systemic lupus
				Membranous
				  nephritis

Table 14.2 Categories of antigen triggering some organ based diseases.

with bacteria, fungi or viruses. **Reiter's syndrome** consists of inflammation of the anterior part of the uveal tract, conjunctivitis and keratitis and is a complication of gastrointestinal or urinary tract infection with certain organisms, e.g. chlamydia and salmonella. **Enteric fever** (often called typhoid fever) is caused by the organism, *Salmonella typhi*, but many of the pathological changes occurring in the gut, including ulceration, are the direct consequence of the immune response to this organism. It has recently become clear that infection with *Helicobacter pylori* is a common cause of **chronic gastritis** as well as peptic ulceration and, possibly, gastric cancer.

Untoward responses can also occur when vaccines are used. A vaccine against **respiratory syncytial virus** (RSV) was withdrawn when it was discovered that children who received it experienced a greater degree of lung damage (due to immune complex formation) when they subsequently contracted the natural infection. The first **measles** vaccine to be introduced was a heat-inactivated preparation but this gave rise to an unusually severe and atypical form of measles following natural infection and was withdrawn in favour of the current live attenuated vaccine which does not have this effect.

Responses to non-microbial antigens

The contribution of the immune response to the development of inflammation and the destruction of body tissues is clearly demonstrated when non-microbial antigens (also called **allergens**) are studied. Their ability to induce dramatic responses was first highlighted at the beginning of this century in two classical descriptions. In the first instance, two French scientists, Portier and Richet, observed that an extract of sea anemone could be safely injected into dogs on a first occasion but induced a severe and fatal reaction when reinjected several weeks later. This adverse reaction took the form of cardiovascular and respiratory collapse and was given the term 'anaphylaxis' to contrast with the protection induced by prophylaxis. It is now known to be mediated by IgE, mast cells and their mediators (see Chapter 15). The second observation was made by two German scientists, Von Pirquet and Schick, who were using hyperimmune horse serum to treat the life-threatening infection, diphtheria. They, too, found that an initial injection was usually uneventful but a fever, rash, joint pains and renal damage often developed about 8 days after a subsequent injection of horse serum. This became known as 'serum sickness' and is now known to be mediated by circulating immune complexes (see Chapter 15).

The term '**allergy**' was initially used to describe any form of altered reactivity that followed exposure to antigenic material but currently is most often used to refer to the symptoms and signs that accompany adverse reactions to non-microbial antigens. Table 14.3 lists some of the more common examples of such antigens. There is marked variation in individual susceptibility to develop allergic responses and many of these responses fall within the general category of **atopic disease**.

It was first recognized in the 1920s that some individuals, and other members of their families, are particularly prone to develop allergic

ANTIGENS CAUSING ALLERGY

Plant pollens
Fungal proteins
Animal danders
House dust mite proteins
Insect stings
Food proteins
Drugs and chemicals
Metals, e.g. chromium, cobalt and nickel
Vaccines

Table 14.3 Some non-infective materials which can trigger allergic responses.

responses to certain non-microbial antigens. These responses usually express themselves in the skin (**atopic dermatitis**), nose (**allergic rhinitis**), eyes (**allergic conjunctivitis**), lungs (**allergic asthma**) and gut (**food allergy**). The tendency to develop such disorders is known as the **atopic trait** and the underlying abnormality is discussed in Chapter 16. Table 14.2 includes these atopic diseases and some other allergic disorders. **Dermatitis herpetiformis** and **coeliac disease** are two forms of adverse reaction to the protein, gliadin, that is present in wheat: the former condition is a blistering skin disease; the latter is characterized by gastrointestinal malabsorption, and both respond to a gliadin-free diet. Air-borne antigens are a common cause of allergic disease and the size of the antigen-containing particle is a major factor in determining which part of the respiratory tract is involved. Allergic rhinitis is usually associated with particles of more than 15 microns in diameter; allergic asthma is associated with particles of less than 15 microns, and **allergic alveolitis** occurs in response to particles within the range 1–5 microns. The smallest size of particles is often produced by moulds that form on a variety of biological materials, e.g. hay, barley, sugar cane, and cheese (see Table 14.4), and those working in close proximity to these materials (e.g. farmers) are more prone to develop allergic inflammation of their alveoli.

Many kinds of disturbance which have been loosely attributed to 'allergy' have nothing to do with immunological responsiveness and the cardinal features of immune responses (e.g. specificity and memory) should be reviewed (see Chapter 1) when attempting to categorize an adverse reaction as immunological or not. **Favism** is a condition in which haemolytic anaemia and jaundice follow the ingestion of broad beans or

ALLERGIC ALVEOLITIS

Disease	Antigenic material
Farmer's lung	*Micropolyspora faeni* (mouldy hay)
Bird fancier's lung	Avian proteins (bird droppings)
Mushroom worker's lung	Thermophilic actinomycetes (mushroom compost)
Bagassosis	Thermophilic actinomycetes (mouldy sugar cane)
Cheese worker's lung	*Penicillium caseii* (mouldy cheese)
Suberosis	*Penicillium frequentans* (mouldy cork)
Malt worker's disease	*Aspergillus clavatus* (mouldy barley)
Ventilator pneumonitis	Thermophilic actinomycetes (humidifers/air conditioners)

Table 14.4 Examples of allergic alveolitis.

various drugs. It was thought to be an immunological phenomenon until a deficiency of glucose-6-phosphate dehydrogenase was identified within the red cell membrane of susceptible individuals. Another example is the adverse response to aspirin and some other drugs and chemicals experienced by a few patients with asthma. In both instances the lack of chemical specificity was always against an immunological explanation. A now classical confusion is that of the inappropriately termed '**total allergy syndrome**' in which some individuals experiencing a variety of symptoms including dizziness and breathlessness following exposure to many different stimuli were considered to have an immunological problem. Most of the symptoms described are now known to be psychological in origin and mediated by hyperventilation and hypocapnia.

Responses to autoantigens

A century ago, Ehrlich contemplated the prospect of unbridled autoreactivity and gave it the term '**horror autotoxicus**'. The first intimation of the existence of human autoimmune disease was the identification of a red cell autoantibody (haemolysin) in a haematological complication of syphilis (paroxysmal cold haemoglobinuria). Many diverse forms of autoimmune disease have been studied since then and these disorders form a major part of clinical immunological practice.

Table 14.2 lists several examples of autoimmune diseases. **Pemphigus** and **pemphigoid** are two blistering skin disorders which are associated with the presence of autoantibodies that react with epithelial components. In the former, the autoantigen is present in the intercellular substance of the epidermis whereas in the latter it is located at the basement membrane. **Lens-induced uveitis** is a condition in which inflammation of the uveal tract follows the release of lens protein after traumatic damage to the lens. In **keratoconjunctivitis sicca** (or Sjögren's disease) an autoimmune response impairs the function of the lacrimal and salivary glands resulting in dry eyes and a dry mouth. An autoimmune response to the glomerular basement membrane (**anti-GBM disease**), in particular, the α3-chain of type IV collagen, is characteristic of Goodpasture's syndrome and gives rise to a severe proliferative glomerulonephritis and, in some cases, bleeding from the lungs. The latter is caused by the same autoantibody which cross-reacts with the basement membrane in the lung (see Chapter 15). **Pernicious anaemia** is associated with a form of chronic gastritis and is characterized by the presence of several autoantibodies one of which is specific for intrinsic factor normally produced by the gastric mucosa and which is essential for the absorption of vitamin B_{12}. **Systemic lupus erythematosus** is an autoimmune condition that causes damage to several organs including the kidneys. Many of the antibodies present react with native (double-stranded) DNA and the immune complexes that result deposit in parts of the circulation where the fluid is filtered across membranes, e.g. in the glomerulus (see Chapter 15).

The cause of autoimmune disease is still one of the unsolved mysteries of immunology. The normal ability of the immune system to discriminate between self and non-self is achieved by (a) a process whereby self-reactive cells are deleted during development, and (b) the inhibition or regulation of residual self-reactive cells by other cells which suppress them either specifically (e.g. suppressor T cells) or non-specifically (e.g. large granular lymphocytes). Some T lymphocytes escape the censoring process in the thymus by which self-reactive cells are eliminated and **clonal inhibition** is therefore required in addition to **clonal deletion**. B lymphocytes, on the other hand, are not subjected to self-reactive censoring but do not receive a 'go' signal from self-reactive T cells unless the normal immunoregulatory mechanisms have broken down.

INFECTION AS A TRIGGER OF AUTOIMMUNITY

There are often pointers toward microbial or chemical agents that may trigger autoimmune responses and there is considerable individual variation in host susceptibility, which governs the severity and chronicity of these processes (see Chapter 16). The immune response to the protozoan organism, *Trypanosoma cruzi*, which causes **Chagas' disease**, is an interesting example of the way in which autoimmunity can develop during the course of an established infection. Acute infection—in which the parasite can be detected in the blood—is characterized by the presence of fever, muscle pain, enlarged liver, spleen and lymph nodes and, in some cases, inflammatory change in the heart muscle, i.e. myocarditis. Around 10–20 years later these patients often present with chronic disease in which cardiac failure and arrhythmias, on the one hand, and impaired motility and dilatation of the gastrointestinal tract, on the other, are major features. Autoantibodies and T cells from patients with chronic disease show specificity for cardiac and neuronal tissue and their presence is associated with loss of the normal conducting fibres in the heart and the parasympathetic nerve plexuses in the gut. Antigens of *T. cruzi* bind to various host cells spontaneously, and antibodies and T cells reactive with them are able to lyse these host cells. Autoimmune features develop subsequent to this.

There are many other clues to possible microbes that may trigger autoimmune responses, e.g. Coxsackie virus infection and autoimmunity to pancreatic islet cells, and if any infection is at all prolonged it is probably unusual to find no evidence of autoreactivity. It is interesting to speculate that if _Treponema pallidum_ had not been identified as the microbial cause of syphilis early on then much of the pathology present in secondary and tertiary syphilis (which includes the development of various kinds of autoreactivity) might well have been regarded as being due to 'autoimmunity'.

   Autoimmune diseases form a major part of medical practice and some of the more important conditions and their respective autoantigens are listed in Table 14.5. In some instances autoantibodies can have pathological effects, e.g. the anti-receptor antibodies of Graves' disease and myasthenia gravis. In others, tissue damage is largely due to the activities of T cells. In either case, the presence of autoantibodies in the circulation is of considerable value in the serological investigation of these diseases and is achieved by using the techniques described in Chapter 6.

AUTOIMMUNE DISEASES AND THEIR ANTIGENS

Organ-specific

Hashimoto's thyroiditis	Thyroid peroxidase, thyroglobulin
Graves' disease (thyrotoxicosis)	Thyroid-stimulating hormone receptor
Pernicious anaemia	Intrinsic factor
Addison's disease	Zona glomerulosa of adrenal cortex (including 21-hydroxylase)
Type I (insulin-dependent) diabetes	Islet cells (including glutamic acid decarboxylase, insulin)
Myasthenia gravis	Acetylcholine receptor
Multiple sclerosis	Myelin sheath of nerve fibres (including myelin basic protein)
Pemphigus	Intercellular substance of epidermis (including desmoglein 3)
Pemphigoid	Epidermal basement membrane
Goodpasture's disease	Glomerular and alveolar basement membranes (including α-3 chain of type IV collagen)
Primary biliary cirrhosis	Mitochondrial enzymes

Systemic

Systemic lupus erythematosus	Double-stranded (native) DNA, ribonucleoprotein
Mixed connective tissue disease	Ribonucleoprotein
Systemic sclerosis	Nucleoli (including topoisomerase)
Dermatomyositis	Aminoacyl tRNA synthetases
Rheumatoid arthritis	IgG

Table 14.5 Some autoimmune diseases and their typical autoantigens.

MECHANISMS OF INDUCTION OF AUTOIMMUNITY

The various mechanisms which have been proposed fall into two main categories: ways in which unreactive T cells can be bypassed and ways in which autoreactive T cells can be stimulated (Table 14.6). Bypassing the requirement for self-reactive T cells does, however, only provide a means of generating autoantibodies and cannot, of itself, produce autoreactive T cells.

Various agents, e.g. endotoxin and Epstein–Barr virus, can act as **polyclonal B cell stimulators** without a requirement for T cell help and this is probably why autoantibodies appear transiently during the course of infectious mononucleosis. Some microbes contain sequences that consist of repeating determinants, e.g. lipopolysaccharide, and thus may be able to function as **T-independent B cell autoantigens**. Some forms of monoclonal B cell proliferation also display autoreactivity (see Chapter 17).

There is now good evidence that, during the immune response to a foreign antigen (epitope), a second wave of antibodies appears which reacts with the **idiotype** of the initial antibody (see p. 82). The idiotype presents a complementary shape to that of the antigenic epitope and thus one would expect the binding sites of some **anti-idiotype antibodies** to show similarity with the original epitope (Fig. 14.2). If, for example, the antigen is a viral component which binds to host cell components, then a proportion of the anti-idiotype antibodies may also bind to the virus receptors and appear as 'autoantibodies'. Anti-idiotype antibodies reactive with reovirus antibody have been shown to bind host cells and mimic or inhibit binding of the virus to these cells. This mechanism may help to explain why so many autoantibodies are directed to structures with

INDUCTION OF AUTOIMMUNITY

Bypassing unreactive T cells
Polyclonal or monoclonal B cell stimulation
T-independent autoantigens
Anti-idiotype reactivity
The carrier effect

Stimulating autoreactive T cells
Molecular mimicry
Impaired immunoregulation
Inappropriate HLA class II expression
Release of sequestered antigen

Table 14.6 Possible ways of inducing autoimmunity.

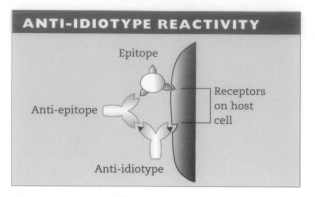

Fig. 14.2 How anti-idiotype reactivity can manifest itself as autoimmunity. For example, the epitope could be a viral component and the anti-idiotype might therefore bind to the virus receptor.

which viruses combine, e.g. DNA, ribonucleoprotein and various RNA fragments and enzymes, and why so many of the antibodies that develop during infection are not specific for the infecting organism. There is, however, little direct evidence for this mechanism operating in human autoimmune disease although several animal models support such a possibility.

The **carrier effect** (Fig. 14.3) enables autoreactive B cells to receive T cell help when a foreign determinant, e.g. drug or virus, becomes covalently linked to a self-determinant. The helper T cells that recognize the foreign determinant can then cooperate with self-reactive B cells to cause them to proliferate and produce autoantibody. Various experimental examples of this phenomenon have been studied and this process is thought to underly the autoimmune haemolytic anaemia that develops following the administration of the drug α-methyldopa or during infection with *Mycoplasma pneumoniae*. These foreign materials become intimately associated with the red cell membrane.

Molecular mimicry describes the situation whereby a pathogenic organism contains a chemical determinant which exactly mimics a component of self. For example, rheumatic fever is a condition in which cardiac inflammation follows streptococcal infection and molecular mimicry has been invoked to explain the presence of antibodies reactive with cardiac muscle which cross-react with components of streptococci. Sequence similarities between microbial proteins and human host proteins can be identified, although many of these similarities are not associated with detectable autoreactivity to the human proteins. Indeed, it is possible that mimicry has a functional value for pathogenic microorgan-

THE CARRIER EFFECT

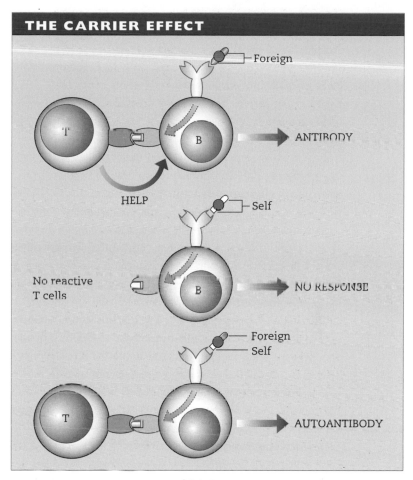

Fig. 14.3 The carrier effect by which T cells reactive with foreign determinants can provide help for self-reactive B cells in the presence of covalently linked 'self' and 'foreign' determinants.

isms as they seek to evade the destructive effect of the immune response by taking advantage of the immunological tolerance of the host to its self-determinants. Sequence homology between a ribosomal protein of *Trypanosoma cruzi* and the human β_1-adrenergic receptor may be relevant to the development of autoimmune myocardial injury in Chagas' disease. Molecular mimicry may be restricted to the B cell compartment with non-homologous microbial determinants stimulating helper T cells (as in the 'carrier effect' described above), or it could involve the stimulation of cross-reactive T cells as well. A reason why autoreactive T cells may be stimulated initially by cross-reactive foreign antigens, but not by the autoantigens themselves, may depend on the way in which the antigens are presented, i.e. their immunogenicity. There is evidence that the immune system maintains **self-ignorance** to many potential auto-antigens because they are not presented by 'professional' antigen presenting cells (i.e. dendritic cells and macrophages) which express HLA class II and costimulatory adhesion molecules (see Chapter 4). By contrast, foreign antigens are normally presented in this way and, once activated by them, T cells may react against cross-reactive autoantigens.

The fact that some individuals and their families are inordinately prone to a variety of autoimmune disorders suggests that **impaired immunoregulation** may underly their susceptibility. The exact identity and role of suppressor T cells in man are ill-defined but various studies suggest that failure to control autoreactive helper T cells is of major importance in some autoimmune disorders. In particular, it may be critical in determining whether an autoimmune response is chronic or short-lived. Studies in mice demonstrate that red cell autoantibodies can be readily induced by injecting the red cells of another species. The autoimmune response declines promptly in normal animals due to the presence of suppressor cells in contrast to animals prone to develop spontaneous autoimmune disease, e.g. the NZB/NZW hybrid mice. The increased prevalence of autoimmune phenomena in various forms of immunodeficiency also lends support to this possibility. As discussed in Chapters 3 and 5, some T cells can inhibit others via the cytokines they secrete. Many autoimmune diseases involve inflammatory T_H1 cells and these may respond unchecked if there is inadequate activation of T_H2 cells which are a source of the T_H1-inhibitory cytokines: IL-4 and IL-10. Restoration of immunoregulation is being attempted in some auto-immune diseases by feeding relevant autoantigens to affected individuals: this exposure to antigens via a mucosal route activates specific T cells which produce suppressive cytokines like IL-4 and transforming growth factor-β.

Class II glycoproteins of the HLA system (see Chapter 2) are normally only expressed on antigen presenting cells, e.g. macrophages and dendritic cells, and B lymphocytes. There is some expression by other cell types including endothelium and cells lining the bronchi and small intestine. **Class II expression** has, however, been described on cells from tissues in which autoimmune disease has become established, e.g. thyrocytes in thyroiditis, pancreatic islets in type I diabetes and liver cells in biliary cirrhosis. It has been proposed that this stimulates autoreactive helper T cells to induce autoreactive cytotoxic T cells and B lymphocytes and ongoing autoimmune destruction. This could, conceivably, have survival value in enabling the host to eliminate persistent viruses within host cells. The antigen presenting capacity of cells like thyrocytes is further supported by their ability to express the adhesion molecule ICAM-1 and to generate IL-1 as a second signal for helper T cell stimulation. However, class II expression is a feature of most infective foci and sites of inflammatory damage, and is possibly a secondary rather than a primary phenomenon; it may even have a role in inducing suppression as the immune response gets under way.

Lastly, self components that do not make contact with the cells of the immune system during development will not be regarded as 'self'. If material containing such components is released during adult life from a site in which it has been sequestered then a vigorous immune response will ensue and will be regarded as autoimmune. Lens protein and sperm antigens have been placed in this category to explain the development of lens-induced uveitis and mumps orchitis, respectively, although it is by no means clear how many other kinds of autoimmune disease can be explained by the **release of sequestered antigen**.

A similar phenomenon may occur at the level of individual epitopes which are not normally presented to the immune system and can be regarded as cryptic self-determinants. The immune system is tolerant of dominant determinants of the same autoantigens, but not to the cryptic epitopes to which a response can occur if they are inadvertently presented in an immunogenic form.

In most situations, it is likely that autoimmune disease arises due to combinations of the processes listed in Table 14.6, e.g. molecular mimicry is unlikely to wreak havoc in the absence of other assistance such as class II expression, and immunoregulatory impairment will become apparent when other forces, such as the development of cross-reactive idiotypes, stimulate the production of autoreactive specificities. Transient autoimmune phenomena are extremely common in infectious disease and after the administration of some drugs and chemical agents. What is not clear is why some patients present with severe and intractable autoimmune disturbances which can be resistant to the most powerful immunosuppressive drugs.

Autoreactive T cells have recently been identified and isolated from patients with autoimmune disease and studies using such cell lines should provide valuable information concerning ways in which the activity of these cells is regulated. The fact that they can be obtained from animals who have recovered from an autoimmune disease suggests that their active suppression is a normal state of affairs.

The subdued but specific ability of the immune system to recognize self-components is undoubtedly an important attribute, e.g. recognition of self-HLA glycoproteins and recognition of self-idiotypes, and is in keeping with the specialization of the immune system from innate properties of intercellular recognition. Thus, autoreactivity may have greater physiological importance than was at first thought and should only be considered as untoward when expressed as the destructive lesions of autoimmune disease.

Responses to unidentified antigens

Although much is known about the nature and identity of antigens triggering human immune responses there is still a long list of serious, and often chronic, diseases which are immunologically mediated but for which the key antigens have yet to be identified. A few examples are included in Table 14.2. There are many forms of inflammation that affect blood vessels, i.e. **vasculitis**, and many of them produce changes in the skin as well as other organs. One example is polyarteritis nodosa and, although a very small proportion of cases have been found to be due to infection with hepatitis B virus, the cause of the remainder is obscure. Henoch–Schonlein purpura is another variant in which the predominant immunoglobulin involved is IgA suggesting that the immune response originates in the gastrointestinal tract. The nature of the stimulus in most forms of **uveitis** is still unknown. This condition usually affects *either* the anterior (iris and ciliary body) or posterior (choroid) part of the uveal tract and can show a histological appearance typical of *either* an immune complex-mediated or cell-mediated form of tissue damage (see Chapter 15); it is likely, therefore, that several causal agents are responsible. **Nasal polyps** cause obstruction of the nasal airway and can be a sequel to long-standing allergic rhinitis. However, in most cases the cause is unknown and the histological features resemble asthma rather than allergic rhinitis. **Pulmonary eosinophilia** is characterized by infiltration of the lung with eosinophils and a raised blood eosinophil count. World-wide, the commonest form is that of tropical eosinophilia which is a sequel to infection with helminths but the mechanism responsible for cases arising in other parts of the world is unclear. **Sarcoidosis** has a similar histological appearance to tuberculosis but without the presence of recognizable mycobacteria. Several studies have reported the detection of nucleotide sequences specific for mycobacteria in sarcoid tissue confirming earlier impressions that this disease represents either an aberrant response to conventional disease-causing mycobacteria or a response to mycobacterial species with unusual growth characteristics.

Crohn's disease is another condition characterized by chronic granulomatous inflammation and usually affects the gastrointestinal tract. Similar studies have been conducted in the search for a microbial cause but with less success, thus far, than in sarcoidosis. There is evidence of acute inflammation in **ulcerative colitis** but the definitive trigger has eluded detailed study so far. **Membranous nephritis** is a form of glomerulonephritis characterized by marked signs of immune complex deposition in the kidney (when examined by immunohistochemical techniques). It is still far from clear why certain individuals develop this condition which responds only poorly to conventional therapy.

Despite the many puzzles that remain, a number of previously mysterious diseases have had their microbial causes identified in recent years, e.g. *Borrelia burgdorferi* as the cause of Lyme disease (affecting skin, joints and the brain); *Escherichia coli* 0157 as a cause of haemolytic–uraemic syndrome; *Helicobacter pylori* as a cause of gastrointestinal disease (see above), hepatitis C, D and E viruses as causes of previously obscure cases of liver inflammation, and parvovirus B19 as the cause of a characteristic rash, arthropathy and anaemia (see Chapter 11 and Table 11.2). Those conditions that remain 'orphans', i.e. without an identified trigger for the immune response that ensues, are likely to be resolved in the near future following the development of molecular microbiological techniques to study the 'footprints' of infection (rather than relying on *in vitro* culture) and the application of modern epidemiological techniques to identify risk factors.

Classification of immunological disorders

Use of the term 'idiopathic' (i.e. cause unknown) is becoming a less common feature of modern textbooks of medicine as causative agents are identified in an increasing number of diseases of infective origin. As time goes by, it is likely that many of the conditions which currently fall within categories 3 and 4 (Table 14.2) will transfer to categories 1 and 2. The striking manifestations of autoimmunity that can be observed during conditions which are incontrovertibly triggered by infection suggest that autoimmunity is rarely, if ever, likely to be the *primary* cause of disease but, rather, reflects the complex nature of the interactions between host and parasite. It is possible that autoimmune phenomena may have survival value for the host or they may demonstrate yet another technique by which parasites are able to divert the aggressive intentions of the immune response.

The upshot of this gradual reclassification of immunological disorders brings us back to the view that all four kinds of response represent 'altered reactivity' (the original definition of allergy) to environmental antigens; be they of microbial or non-microbial origin.

KEY POINTS

1 In addition to coping with the complexity of microbial antigens, the immune system is also prone to be activated by antigens of a non-microbial nature, as well as by autoantigens, and also shows evidence of activation in diseases in which the triggering antigens have yet to be identified.

2 Experiments in animals have clearly demonstrated that the severity of the tissue damage and illness experienced in infectious diseases is often due to the vigour of the immune response rather than to toxic factors released from microbes.

3 Allergic disease is common and usually occurs in response to airborne or ingested antigens.

4 Immune responses to autoantigens have been described in many diseases but unrecognized infection is likely to be the triggering event in most examples. Several mechanisms have been proposed to explain this sequence which may, in some instances, represent another mechanism of evasion by the triggering pathogen.

Further reading

Anon. (1989) Self-tolerance and auto-immunity: bridging the gap. *Lancet*, **i**, 649–650.

Holgate S.T. & Church M.K. (1993) *Allergy*. Gower Medical Publishing, London.

Mims C.A. (1995) *The Pathogenesis of Infectious Diseases*, 4th edn. Academic Press, London.

Oliveira D.B.G. & Lachman P.J. (1993) Autoimmunity. In Lachman P.J., Peters D.K., Rosen F.S. & Walport M.J. eds, *Clinical Aspects of Immunology*, 5th edn. Blackwell Scientific Publications, Oxford.

Plotz P.H. (1983) Auto-antibodies as idiotype antibodies to antiviral antibodies. *Lancet*, **ii**, 824–826.

Rose N.R. & Mackay J.R. eds. (1985) *The Auto-immune Diseases*. Academic Press, London.

Wilkinson J.R.W. & Lee T.H. (1993) General anaphylaxis. In Lachman P.J., Peters D.K., Rosen F.S. & Walport M.J. eds, *Clinical Aspects of Immunology*, 5th edn. Blackwell, Scientific Publications, Oxford.

CHAPTER 15

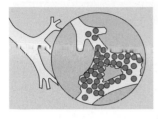

Mechanisms of Immunological Tissue Damage

Whatever the primary cause of a particular immunopathological disorder may be, the mechanisms by which host tissues become damaged belong to four main categories:

1 Reaginic (also called anaphylactic).

2 Cell or membrane-reactive.

3 Immune complex.

4 Cell-mediated.

This classification was originally developed by Coombs and Gell and grew out of the contrasting features of 'immediate' and 'delayed' forms of allergic reaction – often referred to as hypersensitivity. In Table 15.1 (see p. 218) the physiological role of each mechanism is contrasted with pathological examples of each kind of tissue damage. Figure 15.1 illustrates these processes diagrammatically.

Reaginic mechanism

The reaginic or anaphylactic mechanism refers to the events which follow. the combination of antigen with IgE molecules specific for it upon the surface of mast cells. This involves the release of various mediators, e.g. histamine, leukotrienes (LTC$_4$, LTD$_4$, LTE$_4$), chemotactic factors (ECF-A and NCF-A) and platelet activating factor. (PAF), which induce smooth muscle contraction and increase capillary permeability (reviewed in Chapter 9). The physiological value of this process has its origins in antiparasite immunity in which increased vascular permeability promotes the extravascular recruitment of immunological components, e.g. IgG, neutrophils, eosinophils and monocytes, which can then act in concert to inflict damage on the parasite by various forms of lysis. Smooth muscle

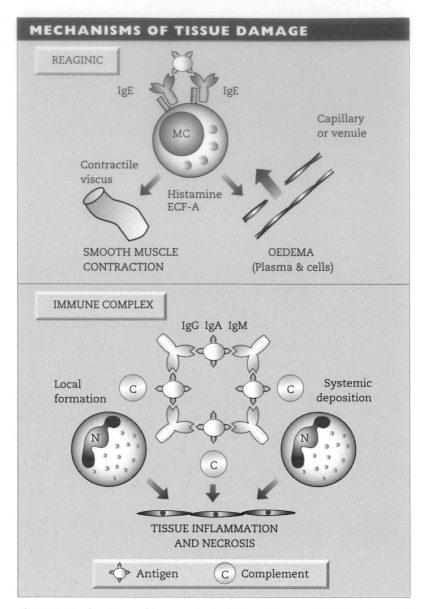

Fig. 15.1 Mechanisms of immunological tissue damage. ECF-A, eosinophil chemotactic factor of anaphylaxis; APC, antigen presenting cell; T_{CP}, cytotoxic precursor T cell; T_H, T helper cell; T_C, cytotoxic T cell; M, macrophage; IL-2, interleukin 2. See text for explanation.

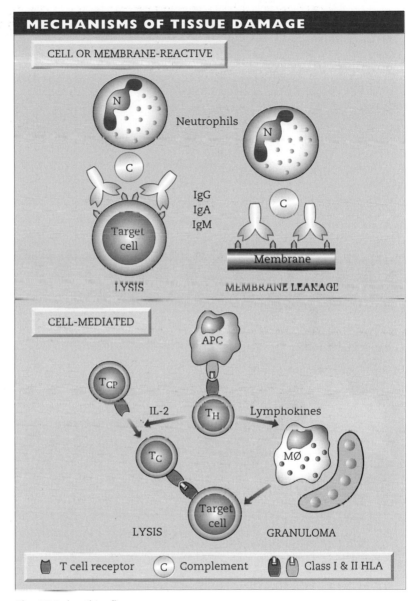

Fig. 15.1 (*continued*)

contraction assists the process and, if it occurs in the gut, can lead to expulsion of the parasite.

Acute **anaphylaxis** is the systemic manifestation of this form of tissue damage and manifests itself as pallor, nausea, hypotension, itching, wheezing, cyanosis, abdominal pain, urticaria and loss of consciousness, all of

CATEGORIES OF TISSUE DAMAGE

Mechanism	Physiology	Pathology	
		Allergic	Autoimmune
Reaginic	Extravascular recruitment of immunological components Parasite expulsion	Anaphylaxis Allergic asthma Allergic rhinitis	?
Cell or membrane reactive	Lysis of pathogens by extracellular or intracellular events	Incompatible blood transfusion Haemolytic disease of the newborn Hyperacute graft rejection	Haemolytic anaemia Thrombocytopenia Pemphigoid Goodpasture's disease Myasthenia gravis* Thyrotoxicosis*
Immune complex	Neutralization of pathogen-derived factors, e.g. toxins Transport of antigen to germinal centres	*Local* Arthus reaction Dermatitis herpetiformis Allergic alveolitis Glomerulonephritis	Rheumatoid arthritis
		Systemic Serum sickness Widespread vasculitis	Systemic lupus Widespread vasculitis
Cell-mediated	Defence against intracellular parasites	Tuberculosis Leprosy Contact dermatitis Graft rejection	Thyroiditis Adrenalitis Pernicious anaemia Diabetes

* The receptor antibodies present in these two conditions have inhibitory or stimulatory effects on the respective receptors rather than complement-mediated lysis.

Table 15.1 The four main categories of tissue damage with examples divided into those known to be triggered by foreign antigens (i.e. allergic) and those deemed to be autoimmune.

which can develop over a remarkably short period of time, e.g. 5–10 minutes. In a susceptible individual, it can follow inoculation by a stinging insect, parenteral administration of an antibiotic, e.g. penicillin, or rupture of a hydatid cyst with release of antigen. Otherwise, pathological effects usually arise as a consequence of IgE produced in response to inhaled or ingested antigens, e.g. pollens, animal danders and foods, and which, in affected individuals, overshadows any previous pre-occupation with antiparasite responses. Reaginic responses express themselves as extrinsic asthma in the lungs, allergic rhinitis in the nose and allergic conjunctivitis in the eyes. These and several other disorders affecting the gut, skin and kidneys fall within the general group of **atopic diseases** (see p. 229).

Autoreactivity mediated by a reaginic mechanism is not well-documented but autoreactive IgE responses could underlie one or other of the conditions characterized by eosinophilia and increased IgE production for which no primary cause has been identified.

Cell or membrane-reactive mechanism

Cell or membrane-reactive tissue damage occurs when specific antibody (of classes IgG, IgA or IgM) combines with antigen on the surface of a cell or basement membrane and which is then able to activate complement and polymorphonuclear leucocytes. Its physiological role is the lysis of pathogens by these extracellular or intracellular processes. Their activity can prove disastrous, however, following an incompatible blood transfusion and during the antibody-mediated 'hyperacute' rejection of tissue grafts. Similar processes are involved in haemolytic disease of the newborn in which maternal antibody reacts with paternal blood group antigens (usually of Rhesus specificity) present on fetal cells.

This mechanism plays a major part in various autoimmune disorders, e.g. autoimmune haemolytic anaemia, idiopathic thrombocytopenic purpura, the bullous skin diseases (e.g. pemphigus and pemphigoid) and Goodpasture's disease (characterized by antiglomerular basement membrane antibodies).

In some autoimmune disorders, antibodies are present which combine with receptors on cell surfaces rather than other target antigens and have metabolic effects rather than causing lytic damage, e.g. anti-acetylcholine receptor antibodies in myasthenia gravis and anti-thyroid-stimulating hormone receptor antibodies in thyrotoxicosis.

Immune complex mechanism

Immune complex-mediated tissue damage is probably the commonest form of all and occurs when soluble antigen combines with soluble antibody. In other words, this form of tissue damage is not confined to the surfaces of cells and can occur locally in a particular tissue or systemically via the circulation. As with the previous mechanism its inflammatory effects follow the activation of complement and phagocytic cells by immunoglobulins of classes IgG, IgA or IgM.

The combination of antibody with microbial toxins and other pathogen-derived factors has an important physiological role in neutralizing their effects and antibody is also of critical importance in transporting antigen to germinal centres in lymphoid tissues to stimulate the recruitment and proliferation of B lymphocytes (see Chapter 4). If local concentrations of antigen become great then an excess of immune complexes will form followed by local tissue damage. This was originally described in the skin as the **Arthus phenomenon** following the repeated injection of heterologous serum. A contemporary example is farmer's lung in which the repeated inhalation of a provoking antigen gives rise to an allergic alveolitis. If excessive amounts of antigen occur in the circulation then immune complexes may deposit systemically. This was first described in the form of **serum sickness** in which a rash, fever, arthritis and glomerulonephritis followed the injection of antidiphtheria horse serum. Similar reactions can follow the administration of drugs and during or following various infections. Immune complex-mediated damage is the basis of poststreptococcal glomerulonephritis, dermatitis herpetiformis, Henoch–Schonlein purpura and other forms of **widespread vasculitis**. Serum sickness-like features occurring in the early phase of viral hepatitis are also due to immune complex formation. This mechanism of damage is also seen in various autoimmune disorders, e.g. locally in joints in rheumatoid arthritis and in many organs in systemic lupus erythematosus.

Cell-mediated mechanism

The cell-mediated mechanism is independent of antibody and occurs when T lymphocytes combine with cell surface antigens. The T cells recruit and activate monocytes and other T lymphocytes (including the precursors of cytotoxic T cells) and generate a powerful inflammatory response with lysis of the target cells. Physiologically, cytotoxic T cells are of particular importance in protection against intracellular parasites, e.g. mycobacteria and budding viruses. This mechanism of tissue damage is prominent in postprimary tuberculosis, leprosy and contact dermatitis and is the more usual means by which foreign grafts are rejected.

The cell-mediated mechanism is one of the slowest to develop and is often referred to as delayed hypersensitivity. The classical cutaneous reaction is usually evident within 24–48 hours but granuloma formation (in which macrophages fuse to form multinucleate giant cells — see Fig. 15.2d) takes at least 14 days. Jones–Mote or cutaneous basophil hypersensitivity is a variant in which the cellular infiltrate contains many basophils and takes 7–10 days to develop, usually in response to soluble antigen. However, basophils or mast cells can be found in classical cell-mediated reactions if the necessary methods of fixation and staining are employed (see p. 122). The organ-specific group of autoimmune diseases, e.g. thyroiditis, adrenalitis, pernicious anaemia and type I diabetes, are all characterized by lymphocytic infiltration and lysis of hormone-producing cells and T cell clones have been derived from such patients which are reactive with organ-specific targets.

Antibody-dependent cell cytotoxicity

Each of the four mechanisms described above require *either* specific antibody *or* T cells for their generation. There is another form of tissue damage which requires the cooperation of both antibody and lymphocyte-like cells, i.e. antibody-dependent cell cytotoxicity (ADCC). Various studies have demonstrated that combinations of IgG antibody and lymphocytes, IgG antibody and monocytes or IgE antibody and monocytes are able to lyse target cells for which the antibody has specificity. Other work shows that eosinophils can also lyse target cells in the presence of IgG or IgE antibody. Some of these events have been alluded to in the preceding discussion concerning the physiological role of the reaginic mechanism. However, it is not yet clear how important this group of mechanisms is in human immunopathology. Large granular lymphocytes are also able to lyse target cells and do not require the presence of specific antibody. As discussed in Chapter 10, these cells overlap with lymphocyte-like cells that mediate ADCC and the role of NK cells in human immunopathology is, as yet, poorly understood.

These different mechanisms have been contrasted with each other for simplicity but it is not uncommon for more than one mechanism to coexist in a particular disease, e.g. injections of immunogenic material can give rise to anaphylactic and serum sickness-like reactions and both

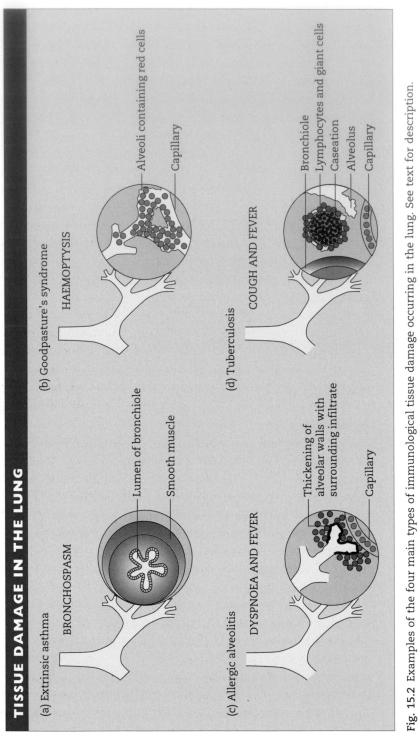

Fig. 15.2 Examples of the four main types of immunological tissue damage occurring in the lung. See text for description.

antibody-mediated and cell-mediated mechanisms have been identified in autoimmune thyroid disease. Attention has also focused on the role of immune complex formation in the lung in allergic asthma (in addition to the reaginic mechanism) and this helps to explain the longer time course of some asthmatic responses to antigen (see below). Unravelling the respective importance of these different processes in particular diseases is one of the challenges of clinical immunology and more detailed information will be found in postgraduate texts.

Clinical examples

LUNG DISEASE

The mechanisms already discussed and their clinical effects are usefully contrasted by taking examples of immunologically mediated tissue damage occurring in the lung (Fig. 15.2).

Extrinsic allergic asthma typifies the reaginic mechanism as exacerbations of this condition are induced when inhaled antigen makes contact with specific IgE on the surface of mucosal and submucosal mast cells, causing their degranulation and release of inflammatory mediators. These mediators cause contraction of bronchial smooth muscle and a degree of bronchial oedema (Fig. 15.2a). Both processes cause narrowing of the airways and intermittent airway obstruction is the hallmark of this condition in contrast to chronic bronchitis and emphysema in which airway obstruction persists.

Maximal reduction in airflow occurs within 10–20 minutes of bronchial challenge with the relevant antigen. A similar latency of response is observed when prick tests are performed in the skin of susceptible subjects. This is in keeping with the earlier description of **immediate hypersensitivity** for the reaginic mechanism. However, a significant proportion of patients with extrinsic asthma show a second and more prolonged fall in airway obstruction several hours after inhalation of antigen. These changes are mediated by IgG, complement and neutrophils and thus involve an immune complex mechanism. This helps to explain why nocturnal asthma can be troublesome after daytime exposure.

A pulmonary example of the cell or membrane-reactive mechanism is **Goodpasture's syndrome** (Fig. 15.2b) in which auto-antibodies react with an antigen present in both glomerular and pulmonary basement membranes, giving rise to acute proliferative glomerulonephritis and parenchymal lung damage with bleeding from the lungs (haemoptysis); this condition is also referred to as lung purpura with nephritis. Damage to the basement membrane follows attachment of IgG antibody and activation of complement and phagocytic cells, culminating in the leakage of blood across it. Little is known about the cause of this condition although epidemiological evidence points to exposure to petrochemicals which, in susceptible subjects of HLA-DR2 phenotype (Table 16.4), may be followed by the development of antibasement membrane antibodies.

Immune complex-mediated damage is exemplified by **extrinsic allergic alveolitis** in which IgG antibody is produced with specificity for inhaled antigen (Fig. 15.2c). The classical example is farmer's lung in which the antigen is a component of spores found in mouldy hay (and see Table 14.4). IgG antibody complexes with antigen across the alveolar–capillary membrane, followed by complement fixation and activation of neutrophils. Clinically, this is manifest as breathlessness (dyspnoea), cough and fever occurring several hours after challenge and a similar latency is observed when skin tests are performed with the appropriate material. This led to the designation of **intermediate hypersensitivity** in contrast to the more rapid immediate form. The dyspnoea which follows acute exposure is due to a decrease in gas transfer across the alveolar–capillary membrane with reduction in the oxygen content of arterial blood. Wheezing or airway obstruction is not a feature of this condition. The proportions of inspired air to perfused blood present in different parts of the lung vary largely due to the effects of gravity on the circulation. In the upright position, the ventilation/perfusion ratio is high in the upper lobes of the lung and low in the lower lobes. Thus the changes of extrinsic allergic alveolitis are more commonly seen in the upper lobes whereas those of the intrinsic form are more commonly found in the lower zones.

Intrinsic (cryptogenic) alveolitis arises as a consequence of the deposition of blood-borne immune complexes in the pulmonary circulation, where they also cause complement and phagocyte activation within the alveolar–capillary membrane. This condition has a more insidious onset without evidence of acute exacerbation but produces similar effects on gas transfer. It often occurs in association with other autoimmune diseases, e.g. rheumatoid arthritis.

Pulmonary tuberculosis and **sarcoidosis** are examples of cell-mediated pulmonary damage. The former follows the inhalation of *Mycobacterium tuberculosis* and usually occurs in the upper lobes, whereas sarcoidosis is usually a more diffuse condition. Primary exposure to *M. tuberculosis* causes a small peripheral focus of infection (the Ghon focus) but with associated enlargement of the lymph nodes at the root of the lung. The primary focus usually heals without symptoms developing and it is only following subsequent (in this context usually referred to as 'post-primary') infection that severe damage to parenchymal pulmonary tissue develops in the upper zones of the lung (Fig. 15.2d). These changes follow activation of various subpopulations of T lymphocytes and the recruitment of macrophages as they respond vigorously to the reintroduced mycobacteria. The involvement and recruitment of both lymphocytes and macrophages is probably why the tempo of this mechanism is the slowest of all and is often referred to as **delayed hypersensitivity**. An equivalent reaction takes place in the skin when sensitized subjects receive an intradermal injection of a mycobacterial extract as in the Heaf, Mantoux or Tine tests. A positive response is characterized by erythema, induration and itching occurring maximally 24–48 hours after challenge.

The intensity of the inflammatory response is such that, in the centre of a lesion, lung tissue is replaced by cheese-like 'caseous' material often with the formation of cavities, which eventually become sealed off by fibrosis and calcification. It was only following the introduction of effective antituberculous drugs that this condition (previously called 'consumption') lost much of its notoriety. The efficacy of some of the more successful agents, e.g. rifampicin, is due, at least in part, to an immunosuppressive effect.

The skin and kidneys are also involved in immunopathological disorders and Fig. 15.3 contrasts examples of membrane-reactive and immune complex damage in these two organs. The bullous or blistering skin diseases, on the one hand, and various forms of glomerulonephritis, on the other, demonstrate how relatively subtle variations in the mechanism and locus of an immunopathological disorder can produce major differences in clinical effects.

SKIN DISEASE

Pemphigus and **pemphigoid** are both caused by circulating auto-antibody reactive with cutaneous antigen. In the former the antigen forms part of the intercellular substance (ICS) of the epidermis and the interaction of IgG auto-antibody with it gives a typical 'chicken wire' pattern of staining on immunofluorescent examination of the skin (Fig. 15.3a). Complement fixation and disruption of the ICS leads to intra-epidermal blister formation. In pemphigoid, the antigen is a component of the epidermal basement membrane and immunofluorescent examination for IgG shows linear staining of this structure (Fig. 15.3b). Subepidermal blister formation follows complement activation at that site. **Dermatitis herpetiformis** is a bullous disorder in which IgA-containing immune complexes deposit in the papillary capillaries (Fig. 15.3d). These activate the alternative complement pathway in the dermal

TISSUE DAMAGE IN SKIN (a–d) & KIDNEY (e–g)

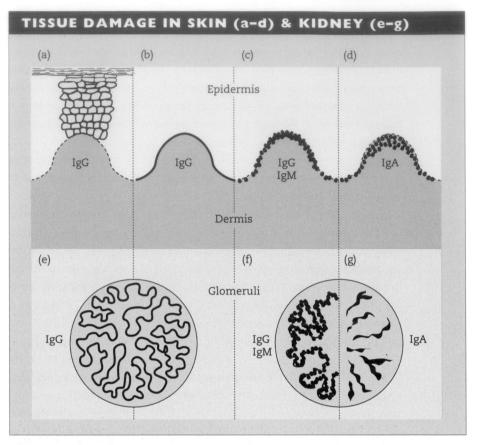

Fig. 15.3 Examples of immunological tissue damage in skin (a–d) and kidney (e–g). (a) Pemphigus; (b) pemphigoid; (c) systemic lupus; (d) dermatitis herpetiformis; (e) Goodpasture's disease; (f) systemic lupus; (g) IgA nephropathy.

papillae and cause subepidermal blister formation. In **systemic lupus erythematosus** (SLE) IgG-containing immune complexes are found beneath the basement membrane of the epidermis (Fig. 15.3c) and although this may be associated with an erythematous rash this does not cause blisters to form.

KIDNEY DISEASE

In **Goodpasture's disease** auto-antibody to the glomerular basement membrane (GBM) can be detected by the presence of diffuse linear staining of the GBM on immunofluorescent examination (Fig. 15.3e). It usually causes an acute proliferative glomerulonephritis with reduced urine production (oliguria), blood in the urine (haematuria) and failure of the clearance function of the kidney (uraemia). Complement activation and infiltration by neutrophil polymorphs are pronounced features of this condition. Immune complex-mediated damage to the glomerulus takes many forms. Diffuse granular deposition of immune complexes containing most classes of immunoglobulin occurs in **SLE** (Fig. 15.3f) and thickening of the basement membrane as well as some degree of proliferative change is usually found in association with marked protein loss in the urine (proteinuria) and uraemia. In **IgA nephropathy** (Berger's disease), IgA-containing complexes preferentially localize in the mesangium of the glomerulus with relative sparing of the basement membrane, giving a radial pattern of deposition (Fig. 15.3g). The clinical features may range from haematuria and proteinuria to no clinical disturbance whatsoever. In some forms of immune complex deposition in the kidney, e.g. **membranous glomerulonephritis**, complexes localize in a subendothelial position where they are least able to recruit neutrophil polymorphs but give rise to considerable thickening of the basement membrane and marked proteinuria.

These examples have been selected to illustrate different patterns of immunologically mediated tissue damage in selected organs. More detailed descriptions of these and other disorders will be found in postgraduate texts.

KEY POINTS

1 The mechanisms of immunologically mediated tissue damage are classified into four main types: reaginic or anaphylactic, cell or membrane-reactive, immune complex, and cell mediated. More than one mechanism may operate in a single disease.

2 The reaginic mechanism involves IgE, mast cells and their mediators (including histamine, leukotrienes and chemotactic factors) which give rise to oedema and smooth muscle contraction. Clinical examples include acute anaphylaxis and allergic asthma.

3 The cell or membrane-reactive mechanism involves IgG, IgA or IgM molecules which, after complexing with antigens on the surface of cells or basement membranes, activate complement and phagocytes resulting in lysis or inflammatory change. Clinical examples include various forms of haemolytic disease, pemphigoid and Goodpasture's disease.

4 The immune complex mechanism involves the combination of soluble antigens with soluble immunoglobulins in the circulation or extracellular fluid followed by deposition of the complexes and activation of complement and phagocytic cells. Clinical examples

Continued on p. 228

KEY POINTS

include the Arthus phenomenon, allergic alveolitis, serum sickness and widespread vasculitis.

5 The cell-mediated mechanism involves T cells and macrophages. It has also been called delayed hypersensitivity as its effects develop more slowly. Clinical examples include: tuberculosis, pernicious anaemia and graft rejection.

6 Immunoglobulins may also work in concert with various kinds of lymphocyte and monocyte to mediate antibody-dependent cell cytotoxicity although its relative importance in many diseases is not yet clear.

Further reading

Chapel H. & Haeney M. (1993) *Essentials of Clinical Immunology*, 3rd edn. Blackwell Scientific Publications, Oxford.

Cohen S., Ward P.A. & McCluskey R.T. (1979) *Mechanisms of Immunopathology*. John Wiley, New York.

Wells J.V. & Nelson D.S. (1986) *Clinical Immunology Illustrated*. Williams and Wilkins, Baltimore.

CHAPTER 16

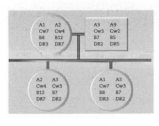

Susceptibility to Immunological Disease

The number of diseases in which immunological processes have been shown to play an important part has steadily increased in recent years and doctors working in all medical specialties need to be aware of the manifestations of immunological disorders. Selected examples are listed by specialty in Table 16.1.

It is still far from clear why some individuals are prone to develop certain kinds of immunological disease whereas others are spared. There is often evidence in favour of a genetic predisposition which, in conjunction with a particular kind of environmental insult, e.g. infection or chemical challenge, produces the critical interaction leading to disease expression. Well-studied examples include allergic asthma, dermatitis herpetiformis, type 1 diabetes and rheumatoid arthritis.

In this chapter, the nature of individual susceptibility is reviewed under three headings: atopic disorders, immune complex disease, and HLA and disease.

Atopic disorders

Atopic disorders form a significant part of human immunopathology in the Western world occurring in at least 5 per cent of individuals. The **atopic trait** can be defined as the spontaneous tendency for an individual to produce high levels of IgE reacting with one or more common antigens in association with antigen-provoked disorders in which a reaginic mechanism can be identified. Table 16.2 lists some of the more important conditions (also mentioned in Chapter 14) in which there is good evidence for the involvement of IgE antibody, mast cells and their mediators. The physiological role of the reaginic mechanism (described in Chapter 15), is concerned with defence against protozoan and metazoan parasites most of which, e.g. plasmodia, schistosomes and trypano-

IMMUNOLOGICALLY MEDIATED DISEASES

Medical specialty	Disease
Cardiology	Rheumatic carditis, cardiomyopathy, postcardiotomy/postinfarction syndromes
Respiratory medicine	Extrinsic and intrinsic alveolitis, extrinsic asthma
Dermatology	Bullous skin disorders, angio-oedema, contact dermatitis
Endocrinology	Addison's disease, type I diabetes, thyroiditis
ENT	Allergic rhinitis, secretory otitis media
Gut and liver	Coeliac disease, ulcerative colitis, acute and chronic hepatitis
Haematology	Autoimmune haemolytic anaemia, neutropenia and thrombocytopenia, pernicious anaemia
Infectious and tropical diseases	Tuberculosis (granuloma), Chagas' disease (myocarditis), malaria (anaemia, nephrotic syndrome)
Obstetrics and gynaecology	Rhesus disease, infertility
Ophthalmology	Allergic/vernal conjunctivitis, uveitis, keratoconjunctivitis sicca
Nephrology	Glomerulonephritis, e.g. poststreptococcal, shunt, bacterial endocarditis, Goodpasture's disease, mesangiocapillary, serum sickness, systemic lupus erythematosus
Neurology	Polymyositis, polyneuritis, multiple sclerosis, myasthenia gravis, postinfective/postimmunization encephalitis
Paediatrics	Atopic eczema, milk and food allergy, juvenile chronic arthritis, Henoch–Schönlein purpura
Rheumatology	Rheumatoid arthritis, systemic lupus, dermatomyositis, widespread vasculitis

Table 16.1 Selected examples of immunologically mediated disease. (From *Lancet*, 1983, ii, 721, with permission.)

ATOPIC DISORDERS

Extrinsic allergic asthma
Allergic rhinitis
Atopic dermatitis
Allergic gastroenteropathy
Seasonal nephrotic syndrome

Table 16.2 Atopic disorders.

somes are now rarely experienced in the Western world. Parasite killing by IgE plus monocytes, eosinophils, platelets or mast cells, or IgG plus eosinophils (the last recruited following ECF-A release by IgE-sensitized mast cells) have each been identified in recent years. The itching, scratching, hypersecretion, sneezing, coughing and contraction of smooth muscle which follows mast cell degranulation is also likely to be of considerable value in effecting the physical removal of parasites and their vectors.

The process of civilization has led to a progressive decline in parasite load and the introduction of novel environments associated with warm houses, modern diets (including formula feeding of infants), high pollen exposure and the keeping of pets, has led to frequent contact with antigens by inhalation or ingestion. This has been associated with a considerable reduction in total and parasite-specific levels of IgE and, thus, Fc receptors on mast cells tend to become preoccupied with IgE molecules with specificity for environmental antigens which do not constitute an infective threat to the host organism. Genetic factors play an important part in determining susceptibility to atopic disease and individuals bearing the HLA A1, B8, DR3 haplotype are more prone to develop allergic asthma and often in association with other atopic disorders as well.

NATURE OF THE DEFECT

Figure 16.1 summarizes the possible locations for the primary defect in atopic disease. The restricted molecular weight range of atopic antigens (25 000–45 000 daltons) might suggest that abnormal mucosal permeability could be a factor but this now seems unlikely. IgA is the usual protective antibody at mucosal surfaces and several studies have shown an increased prevalence of IgA deficiency in atopic individuals and their relatives. Genes have been identified which regulate the level of IgE production but recent work has shown that a variant of the gene for the β subunit of the high-affinity Fc receptor for IgE ($Fc_\varepsilon RI$), present on chromosome 11, is strongly associated with the atopic trait when the gene variant is inherited maternally. Other possibilities concern the ease with which mast cells degranulate; variations in the mediators produced; abnormalities of the molecules which inhibit them (e.g. amine oxidase) and, lastly, variation in their effects on endothelial and smooth muscle cells. Earlier reports that the presence of antiglobulins reactive with IgE (i.e. anti-IgE) or antibodies reactive with β_2 adrenergic receptors might be important have received little confirmation.

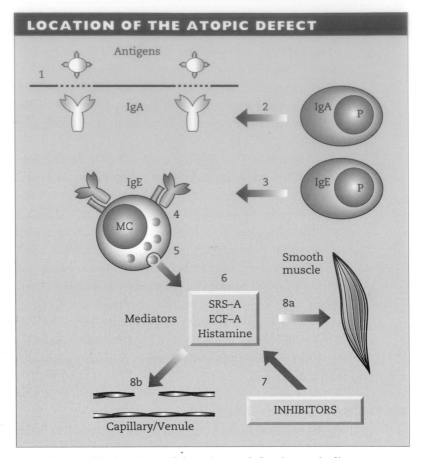

Fig. 16.1 Possible locations of the primary defect in atopic disease.
(1) Abnormal mucosal permeability; (2) impaired IgA production; (3)
increased IgE production; (4) abnormality of the high-affinity IgE receptor
(Fc$_\varepsilon$RI); (5) inappropriate mast cell degranulation; (6) variation in mediator
production; (7) deficiency of mediator inhibitors; (8) (a and b) abnormal
susceptibility of target organs (e.g. smooth muscle and endothelium) to
mediator effects.

Immune complex disease

It is interesting to speculate why some individuals should be particularly
prone to the development of widespread immune complex disease following otherwise straightforward infections. Recently attention has focused on the role of complement components (particularly C4, C2 and
factor B) in maintaining immune complexes in soluble form in body fluids.
Some individuals prone to conditions in which immune complex
mediated damage is a feature, possess genetic variants of these proteins

which are functionally less efficient (see p. 111) and this is probably the major reason why complexes precipitate so readily in these patients and cause an inappropriate degree of tissue damage.

Table 16.3 lists various factors which govern the deposition of immune complexes (IC) within the circulation. Overloading of the normal pathways by which IC are cleared is most likely to occur when there is an excessive quantity or persistence of antigenic material which has sufficient epitope density to form IC of a sufficient size to precipitate (see Fig. 6.9). The isotype (i.e. class and subclass) of the antibodies involved, as well as their affinity of binding, determine their biological effects, and the efficiency of both classical and alternative complement pathways governs how readily IC are solubilized and thus how well they are transported to cells of the mononuclear phagocyte series which are able to ingest and process them. Approximately 1 per cent of the population are heterozygotes for C2 deficiency, and deficiencies of C1q, C1r, C4 and C2 are each associated with a susceptibility to develop immune complex disease (see Chapter 13).

The sites at which circulating IC are deposited are determined partly by their site of formation, e.g. the release of large quantities of antigen from heart valve endothelium in bacterial endocarditis and its combination with circulating antibody give rise to considerable deposition downstream in the kidneys (and other organs which are major recipients of the arterial supply). Turbulence of blood flow and local increases in vascular permeability also affect localization. Immune complexes are often deposited at the various sites at which plasma colloid is filtered to produce other body fluids, e.g. renal glomeruli, choroid plexus, synovium, epidermal basement membrane and uveal tract. An aggregation/concentration effect occurs as soluble complexes pass across these semipermeable membranes and this is why the localization of circulating IC may

FACTORS AFFECTING IC DEPOSITION

Antigen quantity and persistence
Antibody isotype and affinity
Solubilization capacity of serum (C1, C4, C2)
Local factors
  Site of immune complex formation
  Turbulence
  Capillary permeability
  Filtration effects

Table 16.3 Factors governing the deposition of circulating immune complexes.

appear to be confined to a single location and in a subepithelial position, e.g. as in membranous glomerulonephritis.

The formation of soluble IC has an important physiological role and it is only when their formation or clearance become grossly disturbed that the manifestations of 'immune complex disease' become of clinical concern.

HLA and disease

Initially, HLA typing was mainly performed to determine the degree of compatibility between donors and recipients prior to organ transplantation. However, it was soon realized that the presence of certain HLA types (often called 'antigens' because they have been defined by using antibodies specific for them) was positively associated with particular diseases (see Table 16.4). For many years serological typing (using a technique known as microlymphocytotoxicity) was only applicable to the HLA-A and HLA-B series of antigens (see p. 33) and thus the first disease

HLA TYPES AND DISEASE

Disease	HLA type	Frequency (%) Patients	Frequency (%) Controls	Relative risk	Aetiological fraction
Idiopathic haemochromatosis	A3	76	28.2	8.2	0.67
Congenital adrenal hyperplasia	B47	9	0.6	15.4	0.08
Ankylosing spondylitis	B27	90	9.4	87.4	0.89
Dermatitis herpetiformis	DR3	85	26.3	15.4	0.80
Coeliac disease	DR3	79	26.3	10.8	0.72
Sicca syndrome	DR3	78	26.3	9.7	0.70
Graves' disease	DR3	56	26.3	3.7	0.42
Type I diabetes	DR3	56	28.2	3.3	0.39
Type I diabetes	DR4	75	32.2	6.4	0.63
Systemic lupus	DR3	70	28.2	5.8	0.58
Membranous nephropathy	DR3	75	20.0	12.0	0.69
Multiple sclerosis	DR2	59	25.8	4.1	0.45
Narcolepsy	DR2	100	21.5	135.0	1.0
Goodpasture's syndrome	DR2	88	32.0	15.9	0.82
Rheumatoid arthritis	DR4	50	19.4	4.2	0.38
Hashimoto's thyroiditis	DR5	19	6.9	3.2	0.13
Pernicious anaemia	DR5	25	5.8	5.4	0.20

Table 16.4 Some examples of associations between HLA types and disease. (After Svejgaard et al. (1983) Immunological Reviews, **70**, 193–218.)

associations described were with variants at these loci, e.g. ankylosing spondylitis (B27) and haemochromatosis (A3). Many other A and B locus associations were described but when serological typing became possible for D locus antigens, i.e. DR typing, it was realized that many HLA-associated diseases, e.g. type I diabetes, coeliac disease and rheumatoid arthritis, were more strongly associated with DR variants. The diseases listed in Table 16.4 are only a selection of those that have been described in the literature.

B locus associations are often with diseases which are not of an immunological nature, whereas most of the conditions which are closely related to D locus variations are diseases in which immunological processes play an important part and this may give a clue to the underlying mechanism of association (see below). Some disorders e.g. type I diabetes and coeliac disease, show association with more than one DR antigen and, in the former case, individuals heterozygous for the two antigens, i.e. who are DR3/DR4, are at greater risk than those homozygous for either DR3 or DR4, suggesting the presence of two different susceptibility genes or the formation of a novel class II heterodimer (see p. 31).

In view of the critical requirement for these polymorphic HLA glycoproteins to present antigenic peptides to helper T cells when an immune response is triggered, one would expect variations between HLA types to be associated with marked differences in the outcome of infectious diseases. A recent study performed in West Africa has shown a strong association between HLA B53 and resistance to severe malaria which is probably mediated by a heightened immune response to an antigen expressed during the liver stage of malarial infection. There is a need for more work on the relationship between HLA genotypes and the response to infectious agents as, until now, most studies have been concerned with non-infective disorders prevalent in Western environments.

MEASURING THE STRENGTH OF ASSOCIATIONS

There are various ways of estimating the strength of these associations (see Table 16.4). A convenient way to display data obtained for a series of patients and controls with respect to the presence or absence of a particular antigen is in the form of a 2×2 table (Table 16.5). The **relative risk** (RR) is then the cross or odds ratio, i.e. $(a \times d)/(b \times c)$. This value indicates how many times more frequently the disease develops in individuals positive for this antigen compared to individuals who lack it. Another estimate is to compute the **aetiological fraction** (AF), i.e. how much a disease is directly due to the disease-associated factor under investigation. This value can only be used when the RR value is greater

DOCUMENTING ASSOCIATIONS		
	Number of individuals	
	HLA antigen positive	HLA antigen negative
Patients	a	b
Controls	c	d

Table 16.5 A 2 × 2 table to display data concerning a possible association between the presence of an HLA antigen and the presence or absence of a disease (see text).

than 1 (i.e. for those individuals who have an increased risk) and is determined by the following calculation:

$$AF = \left(\frac{RR - 1}{RR} \right) \left(\frac{a}{a + b} \right)$$

Those associations having a greater relative risk usually also possess a greater aetiological fraction but this is not universally so, for, where a particular gene has a very low frequency in the healthy population and is present in only a minority of patients with the disease, the aetiological fraction will be disproportionately low. An example of this is the possession of B47 which confers a relative risk of congenital adrenal hyperplasia of 15.4 which in Table 16.4 can be seen to be the same as for the association between HLA DR3 and dermatitis herpetiformis whereas the aetiological fractions for these two associations are 0.08 and 0.80, respectively.

The strongest HLA–disease association discovered so far is that between DR2 and narcolepsy giving a relative risk of 135 and an aetiological fraction of 1.0. The magnitude of the latter strongly suggests that HLA-DR2 is intimately involved in the disease process and may be linked to a receptor or neurotransmitter defect.

PHENOTYPES, GENOTYPES AND HAPLOTYPES

In the absence of a significant degree of consanguinity, each individual is likely to possess a different set of HLA genes on paternal and maternal chromosomes. The total set is known as the **phenotype** which can be rewritten as the **genotype** when sufficient other members of the family have been studied to identify which genes belong to which chromosomes

(Fig. 16.2). The collection of particular antigens which are under the control of genes borne on a single chromosome is known as the **haplotype** (e.g. a, b, c or d in Fig. 16.2). HLA haplotypes can be written in even more detail, e.g. the haplotype A1/D0/Cw7/DR3 usually possesses the following alleles at the intervening complement loci: C2C, C4AQO, C4BB1 and BfS so that this becomes (reading from left to right along the short arm of chromosome 6, as depicted in Fig. 2.10) DR3–C4BB1–C4AQO–BfS–C2C–B8–Cw7–A2. This is termed the **extended haplotype**. Even though each of these loci are very polymorphic, and the loci on each chromosome bear one of many possible alleles, certain alleles at one locus, e.g. HLA-A, are found much more often with certain alleles at other loci, e.g. HLA-B. These non-random arrangements are a common occurrence within particular populations and this phenomenon is known as **linkage disequilibrium**.

Until recently, HLA typing was usually performed to determine variations at the HLA-A, B, C and DR loci. These data, obtained using serological techniques, are now augmented by DNA techniques that enable the genes associated with particular specificities to be identified.

Genotype nomenclature

The nomenclature used to describe these more detailed genotypes contains information about the locus (and for class II, which α or β chain)

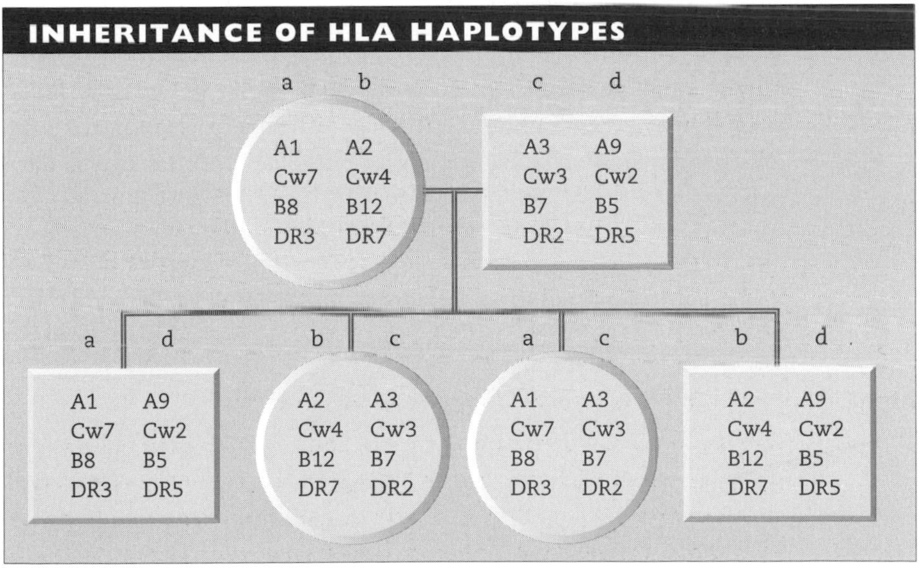

Fig. 16.2 The inheritance of HLA haplotypes. See text.

before an asterisk, followed by numerals assigned to the specificity and gene number, i.e.

For class I: Locus/*/Specificity/Gene number, e.g. A*1102 is the second gene belonging to specificity 11 of the A locus.

For class II: Locus/Chain/*/Specificity/Gene number, e.g. DQA1* 0401 is the first gene belonging to specificity 4 of the first DQ α chain locus whereas DRB3*0201 is the first gene belonging to specificity 2 of the third DR β chain locus.

MECHANISMS OF ASSOCIATION

Several proposals have been made to explain the mechanism of association between HLA types and disease (Table 16.6). Genes controlling specific immune responses were originally characterized in the murine major histocompatibility complex (MHC) and described as **immune response (Ir) genes**. Similar phenomena have been documented in man, e.g. the immune response to ragweed antigen (associated with HLA-Dw2), insulin (associated with HLA-DR7) and streptococcal extracts (associated with HLA-Dw6) and other work favoured the existence of specific immune suppression (Is) genes. It is now clear that the Ir (or Is) genes are the HLA Class II genes themselves by virtue of the differential ability of their $\alpha\beta$ heterodimers on the surface of antigen presenting cells to present antigen (of self or exogenous origin) to T cells. This proposal is supported by the finding that the presence of an arginine residue at position 52 of the DQ α chain and the absence of an aspartic acid residue at position 57 of the DQ β chain are strongly correlated with susceptibility to type I diabetes in Caucasians (with a relative risk of over 40 for homozygotes). Class I associations—of an immunological kind—are likely to be mediated by variation in the way cytotoxic T cells recognize their targets.

MECHANISMS OF ASSOCIATION

Effects of class II polymorphism on antigen presentation
Effects of class I polymorphism on target recognition by cytotoxic T cells
Complement or phagocyte polymorphisms
Molecular mimicry
Receptor interaction

Table 16.6 Mechanisms of association of disease with HLA.

The human MHC also contains four loci coding for important complement components and several of the extended haplotypes known to associate with some of the DR-related diseases contain genes which code for functionally inadequate or absent complement proteins. Individuals bearing certain haplotypes are less able to clear immune complexes from the circulation (see Chapter 7) and show significant differences in phagocyte function. It seems likely that variations in the quality of effector systems such as complement and phagocytic cells, i.e. **complement** or **phagocyte polymorphisms** could be important in determining the outcome of virus infections which may damage host tissues whether an autoimmune response follows or not.

Others have argued that these disease associations occur because of chemical similarity, often called **molecular mimicry**, between the chemistry of these self proteins and chemical determinants present on invading microorganisms (and see p. 207). Much attention has been paid to the relationship between the possession of HLA-B27 and various reactive arthritides, e.g. those which follow infection with organisms belonging to species of *Salmonella*, *Shigella* and *Yersinia*.

Evidence is also accumulating that HLA proteins may intimately associate with hormone and virus receptors on the surface of cells, i.e. **receptor interaction**, and the extremely strong association between DR2 and narcolepsy may be an example of this.

Contributions from other gene loci

Genes coding for structural variations in IgG molecules (the Gm system) and the acute phase protein α-1-antitrypsin (the Pi system) are both present on chromosome 14. These allotypic variations influence susceptibility to a number of diseases and Gm and Pi alleles have been shown to have an interactive effect with HLA alleles in various disorders, e.g. multiple sclerosis, myasthenia gravis and coeliac disease.

Recent developments in DNA technology involving the use of HLA gene probes and endonuclease restriction enzymes have enabled many polymorphisms to be identified within the HLA complex. This approach will enable disease susceptibility or resistance genes to be mapped with greater accuracy and disease associations to be identified even when there is no evidence of association with HLA polymorphisms.

KEY POINTS

1 Doctors working in all medical specialties are confronted by immunologically mediated diseases but the reasons why some individuals are susceptible to particular examples of them are incompletely understood.

2 Atopic diseases occur in at least 5 per cent of individuals in developed countries and include allergic asthma, allergic rhinitis and atopic dermatitis. Evidence has pointed to various possible defects in the handling of environmental antigens or impaired control of mast cell degranulation and recent work suggests that variation in the structure of the IgE Fc receptor may be an important predisposing factor.

3 A number of disorders are caused by the inappropriate deposition of immune complexes. Various factors govern the formation and clearance of immune complexes and the complement system has a critical role in ensuring their solubilization and transport to cells of the mononuclear phagocyte system. Deficiency of certain complement components is often associated with immune complex disease.

4 The HLA type of an individual is a contributory factor toward the susceptibility of many immunological disorders. Most of the studies performed so far have focused on chronic diseases in developed countries but recent work from West Africa demonstrates that the HLA phenotype has a major influence on the outcome of malarial infection. The most likely explanation for these associations is the effect that polymorphism of class I and class II HLA glycoproteins has on T cell cytotoxicity and antigen presentation, respectively. Polymorphism of genes for components of complement and phagocyte function may also play a part.

Further reading

Bell J.I. & McMichael A.J. (1993) Major histocompatibility complex polymorphism in disease susceptibility. In Lachmann P.J., Peters D.K., Rosen F.S. & Walport M.J. eds, *Clinical Aspects of Immunology*, 5th edn. Blackwell Scientific Publications, Oxford.

Devey M.E. & Isenberg D.A. (1988) Immune complex disease – theoretical aspects. In Bird G. & Calvert J.E. eds, *B Lymphocytes in Human Disease*. Oxford University Press, Oxford.

Hopkin J. (1994) Wheeze, sneeze and genes. *Journal of the Royal College of Physicians*, **28**, 560–563.

Lechler R. ed. (1994) *HLA and Disease*. Academic Press, London.

Parham P. (1993) Good news from Gambia. *Current Biology*, **3**, 223–225.

Platts-Mills T.A.E. (1993) The immunobiology of immunoglobulin E: immediate or type I hypersensitivity. In Lachmann P.J., Peters D.K., Rosen F.S. & Walport M.J. eds, *Clinical Aspects of Immunology*, 5th edn. Blackwell Scientific Publications, Oxford.

Reeves W.G. (1984) HLA phenotype and insulin antibody production. *Clinical and Experimental Immunology*, **57**, 443–448.

CHAPTER 17

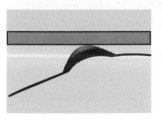

Lymphoproliferative Disease

The study of lymphoid tissue used to be a difficult task in view of the lack of clear and constant structural features and readily distinguishable cell types. Lymphocytes numerically overshadow the other cell types present in lymph nodes and recirculate through the lymphatic system. The delineation of the follicle-containing cortex from the medulla and the identification of specialized postcapillary venules (PCV) at their junction, started the process of understanding the relative roles and cellular constituents of these compartments and their cell traffic patterns (see Fig. 4.6). The development of reagents (e.g. monoclonal antibodies) specific for T and B lymphocytes and their subpopulations and the identification of various kinds of antigen-presenting dendritic cell, in conjunction with *in vivo* studies of lymphocyte traffic patterns, have led to an appreciation of the complex dynamics of lymphoid tissue and the way these processes are perturbed in disease.

Lymphocytosis and lymphadenopathy

The common clinical problems are those associated with an excessive number of lymphocytes in the blood (**lymphocytosis**), enlarged lymph nodes (**lymphadenopathy**) or lymphocytic infiltration of other tissues. These can have many causes, including infection, autoimmune disease and neoplastic disorders. **Leukaemias** are characterized by the presence of abnormal white cells in blood and bone marrow. In **lymphomas** the normal structure of lymphoid tissues is replaced by abnormal cells of lymphoid origin and in some conditions, e.g. chronic lymphocytic leukaemia, both features coexist. Some forms of lymphoproliferative disease, e.g. **myeloma** and **macroglobulinaemia,** are associated with the production of excessive quantities of the secreted products of individual clones of lymphocyte-derived cells and are collectively known as monoclonal gammopathies.

The distinction between the characteristics of peripheral blood lymphocytes and lymphoid tissues (a) in the normal resting state, (b) during antigenic stimulation, and (c) in established lymphoproliferative disease has been greatly facilitated by the use of markers for normal, activated and transformed cell types. These markers include cytogenetic abnormalities; enzyme activities and polymorphisms; immunoglobulin isotypes (e.g. κ vs. λ); cell surface glycoproteins (e.g. HLA and various receptors); and the ability to detect rearrangements in the genes coding for immunoglobulins and the T cell receptor proteins. This powerful armoury not only makes it possible to distinguish the cell type respons-ible for lymphocyte excess or infiltration but also enables the distinction to be made between proliferations which are **monoclonal**, i.e. derived from a single progenitor cell, and those that are **polyclonal**, i.e. derived from a variety of cells.

The three main categories of lymphoproliferative disease, i.e. leukaemias, lymphomas and monoclonal gammopathies, are now re-viewed in turn. In each case, the abnormal proliferation of lymphoid or myeloid cells relates to a physiological counterpart and the particular stage of differentiation involved is indicated in Fig. 17.1.

Viruses and oncogenes

The pathogenesis of lymphoproliferative diseases is poorly understood but the identification of several lymphotropic viruses, e.g. Epstein–Barr (EB) virus, HTLV I and HIV, in association with various kinds of lymphoma and leukaemia, suggests that infection with a virus belonging to this group may be a critical requirement. However, the large majority of EB virus infections, for example, are self-limiting, due to an effective T cell re-sponse and it is probably only when this is deficient, e.g. in chronic malarial infection or in patients with AIDS or other forms of immunodeficiency, that B cell proliferation leads to overt lymphoma (see p. 243).

Cell-transforming or oncogenic RNA viruses contain **oncogenes** (V-onc) which, following the production of DNA transcripts (via reverse transcriptase), are able to alter the proliferative behaviour of the host cell because they code for growth factors, growth factor receptors or their second messengers, e.g. tyrosine kinases. The genome within human cells also contains similar sequences (C-onc) which are normally present in

LYMPHOPROLIFERATIVE DISEASES

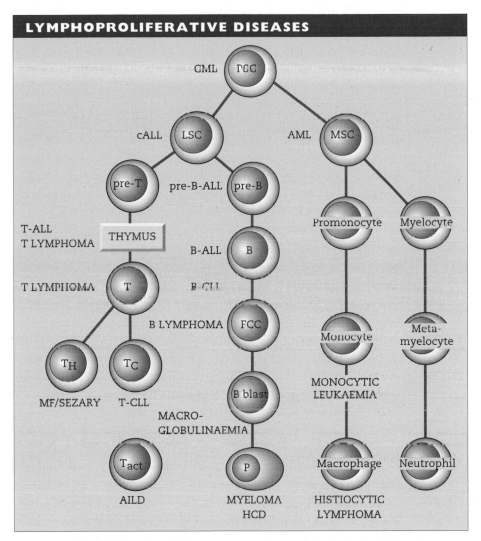

Fig. 17.1 Differentiation pathways of lymphoid and myeloid cells, indicating the cell stages from which lymphoproliferative diseases arise. PSC, pluripotent stem cell; LSC, lymphoid stem cell; MSC, myeloid stem cell; FCC, follicle centre cell; T_{act}, activated T cell; P, plasma cell; CML, chronic myeloid leukaemia; cALL, common acute lymphoblastic leukaemia; AML, acute myeloid leukaemia; MF, mycosis fungoides; CLL, chronic lymphocytic leukaemia; AILD, angio-immunoblastic lymphadenopathy with dysproteinaemia; HCD, heavy chain disease.

latent form (proto-oncogenes). These become activated in particular circumstances, e.g. during embryogenesis or clonal stimulation of lymphocytes. Several of the **chromosomal translocations** found in lymphoproliferative disease are known to affect the expression of host oncogenes, e.g. the transfer of material between chromosomes 8 and 14 in Burkitt's lymphoma, and between chromosomes 9 and 22 which gives rise to the Philadelphia chromosome in chronic myeloid leukaemia. The relationship between infection with oncogenic viruses and the expression of host oncogenes is an area of active investigation.

Epstein–Barr virus and infectious mononucleosis

This common condition is usually self-limiting but has implications for various lymphoproliferative diseases. It occurs when primary infection with **EB virus** is delayed beyond childhood. The virus is spread by saliva and replicates in B lymphocytes. The transformation and proliferation of infected B cells is brought under control by T cells of cytotoxic phenotype which recognize EB virus-determined antigens on the B cell surface. These immunological events coincide with the development of fever, sore throat, lymphadenopathy, splenomegaly and the appearance of **atypical mononuclear cells** (activated T cells) in the peripheral blood. A variety of virus-specific antibodies can be detected as well as the typical heterophil antibody of the Paul–Bunnell test, and some autoantibodies, e.g. red cell and smooth muscle antibodies, occur transiently. After recovery, latently infected B cells are released into the circulation throughout life and are constantly eliminated by cytotoxic T cells.

The **Duncan** or **X-linked lymphoproliferative** (XLP) syndrome is a familial condition in which a defective T cell response fails to control primary EB virus infection, leading to uncontrolled B cell proliferation and the development of lymphoma. As described below, EB virus infection also has a role in the pathogenesis of Burkitt's lymphoma, Hodgkin's disease and non-Hodgkin's lymphomas (as well as nasopharyngeal carcinoma and smooth muscle tumours) but the nature of any genetic susceptibility is still unclear. The development of a vaccine against EB virus is the subject of current research.

Leukaemias

Leukaemia can develop slowly over a period of years or may present abruptly with clinical evidence of bone marrow involvement, e.g. anaemia, bleeding or infection. Leukaemia is designated 'acute' when more than 50 per cent of bone marrow cells are lymphoblasts or myeloblasts.

ACUTE LYMPHOBLASTIC LEUKAEMIA (ALL)

This condition mostly affects children and is classified into five distinct types. Three types arise from B cell precursors; have leukaemic cells that are positive for B cell lineage markers, and show rearrangements of their immunoglobulin genes. They are known as **early B cell precursor ALL** (previously designated 'null'); **common ALL** and **pre-B ALL** (Table 17.1). Common ALL cells are also positive for CD10 (previously referred to as the common ALL antigen – CALLA) whereas pre-B ALL is distinguished by the presence of cytoplasmic immunoglobulin. The cells of each of these B cell precursor types of ALL contain a nuclear enzyme – TdT (see Table 17.1). By contrast, **B ALL** cells are negative for terminal deoxynucleotidyl transferase (TdT) and CD10 but possess surface immunoglobulin. About 15 per cent of ALL are designated **T ALL**. They arise from early thymocytes and their leukaemic cells possess T cell lineage markers and nuclear TdT.

Children with common ALL do well (over a 5-year span) on a regimen of repeated courses of combination chemotherapy. T-ALL and B-ALL are more resistant to cytotoxic agents and have a greater tendency to relapse. Bone marrow transplantation in first or second remission can enhance survival.

CELL MARKERS IN ALL

	B cell lineage						T lineage	Myeloid
	nTdT	CD10	CD19 cCD22	cIg	sIg	Class II	CD7 cCD3	CD13 CD33
Early B cell precursor ALL	+	–	+	–	–	+	–	–
Common ALL	+	+	+	–	–	+	–	–
Pre-B ALL	+	+/–	+	+	–	+	–	–
B ALL	–	–	+	–	+	+	–	–
T ALL	+	–	–	–	–	–	+	–
AML	–	–	–	–	–	–	–	+

nTdT, nuclear terminal deoxynucleotidyl transferase; CD10 was previously known as the common ALL antigen (CALLA); CD19 and cytoplasmic CD22 are B lineage markers; cIg, cytoplasmic immunoglobulin (μ chains); sIg, surface immunoglobulin; Class II, HLA Class II glycoprotein; CD7 and cytoplasmic CD3 are T lineage markers; CD13 and CD33 are myeloid lineage markers.

Table 17.1 Cell markers in acute leukaemia.

ACUTE MYELOBLASTIC LEUKAEMIA (AML)

This occurs at all ages but is the commonest form of leukaemia in adults. It arises following the clonal proliferation of the **myeloid stem cell** (Fig. 17.1), normally the precursor of both monocytes and neutrophils. In AML the blasts usually show some evidence of differentiation to granulocytes, in contrast to ALL in which the blast cells show no differentiation at all. AML cells are positive for myeloid cell markers (e.g. CD13 and CD33), myeloperoxidase and non-specific esterase but are negative for TdT and the markers which characterize T and B cell precursors, including CD10.

Combination chemotherapy is used in AML but remission is more difficult to achieve and marrow failure is more difficult to reverse. Bone marrow transplantation is giving encouraging results in younger patients with AML in first remission although this option largely depends on the availability of a suitable donor.

CHRONIC LYMPHOCYTIC LEUKAEMIA (CLL)

This is a disease of the elderly, it develops insidiously and can remain stable for many years. The circulating lymphocyte count may be 100 times normal and often without symptoms or physical signs. Younger patients have a more active course. Infection complicating secondary antibody deficiency and bone marrow failure are later sequels to which patients usually succumb. CLL does not transform into acute leukaemia but can develop into lymphoma.

In the majority of cases the cell phenotype is that of the mature B cell, i.e. positive for surface immunoglobulin and HLA DR and designated **B-CLL**. In about 10 per cent, a monoclonal immunoglobulin is secreted of the same isotype as that detected on the surface of the CLL cells. Autoimmune haemolytic anaemia and thrombocytopenia occur in a minority. Rare cases are of T cell phenotype and can be CD4$^+$ or CD8$^+$ (**T-CLL**). Cutaneous involvement is common and there is considerable overlap with the Sézary syndrome, mycosis fungoides and T cell lymphomas (see p. 249).

CLL is treated with prednisolone and/or an alkylating agent when there is evidence of bone marrow failure, involvement of lymph nodes or spleen, or autoimmune haemolytic anaemia or thrombocytopenia. Intramuscular or intravenous γ-globulin is an important adjunct in those patients with secondary hypogammaglobulinaemia.

CHRONIC MYELOID LEUKAEMIA (CML)

CML is a disease of middle life but usually presents with symptoms and signs of leukaemic infiltration, e.g. splenomegaly. The blood shows a marked increase in leucocytes (at least fivefold and often much higher). The abnormal cells derive from the **pluripotential stem cell** (Fig. 17.1) and show a cytogenetic abnormality—the **Philadelphia chromosome** — due to translocation of part of the long arm of chromosome 22 to the long arm of chromosome 9 with reciprocal translocation of part of chromosome 9 containing the ABL oncogene to chromosome 22. Most patients develop a blast crisis in which the cell type transforms to give a picture resembling AML or ALL, underlining the common origin of the two cell types concerned.

Most patients with CML respond to treatment with an alkylating agent and splenic irradiation or splenectomy, where necessary. Bone marrow transplantation is being increasingly used in younger patients who have an HLA-matched sibling and this offers the prospect of long-standing remission.

Lymphomas

In these forms of lymphoproliferative disease normal lymphoid tissue is replaced by abnormal cells of lymphoid origin.

HODGKIN'S DISEASE

Hodgkin's disease typically presents in young adults with painless enlargement of regional lymph nodes. Histologically, it is characterized by the presence of large multinucleate cells of irregular shape known as **Reed–Sternberg cells**, which are surrounded by a mixed cellular infiltrate consisting of T and B lymphocytes, macrophages, neutrophils, eosinophils and plasma cells. Systemic symptoms such as fever, anorexia and weight loss are often present, particularly when lymph node involvement has progressed to other sites.

Reed–Sternberg cells are positive for HLA Class II glycoproteins, IgG Fc receptors and the granulocyte marker CD15 but are not phagocytic. They also express the IL-2 receptor (CD25) typical of activated T cells, and the transferrin receptor. It is likely that the Reed–Sternberg cell arises from an early lymphoid cell. Hodgkin's tissue is often positive for the EB virus genome and epidemiological data support a role for EB virus in the pathogenesis of this condition.

Hodgkin's disease is classified histologically into four subtypes: lymphocyte predominant, nodular sclerosis, mixed cellularity and lymphocyte depleted. Nodular sclerosis is distinct from the other three histological subtypes and shows a nodular pattern surrounded by collagen bands. Once this pattern is established it remains constant throughout the course of the disease. The subtype of Hodgkin's disease is important in predicting survival; those with lymphocyte predominant disease have the best survival; mixed cellularity and nodular sclerosis have an intermediate prognosis, and those with lymphocyte depletion have the worst.

Treatment is dependent on the stage of the disease. If it is localized, radiotherapy is the treatment of choice but if further advanced, multiple agent systemic chemotherapy is used. Approximately three-quarters of patients treated for Hodgkin's disease survive for at least 5 years.

NON-HODGKIN'S LYMPHOMAS

The increase in knowledge of the biology of the lymphocyte has led to a greater understanding of the commonest tumours of the immune system — the non-Hodgkin's lymphomas (NHL). This has given rise to more informative classifications of these neoplasms. The Kiel classification has been most widely used and the brief outline given here is based upon it. The majority (>90 per cent) of non-Hodgkin's lymphomas are of the B lymphocyte lineage, 10 per cent are of T cell origin and a small percentage express neither T nor B cell markers and are termed 'null' cells.

There is an increased incidence of NHL in patients with impaired T cell immunity due to therapeutic immunosuppression (given for autoimmune disease or to suppress graft rejection); HIV infection, or inherited deficiencies. EB virus can be detected in most lymphomas occurring in graft recipients. A chromosomal translocation between chromosomes 14 and 18 is present in about 80 per cent of follicular lymphomas. It gives rise to over-expression of the *BCL*-2 oncogene which prevents apoptosis (programmed cell death).

The commonest forms of non-Hodgkin's lymphoma are derived from the germinal centre. In normal lymphoid tissue the germinal centre contains two kinds of **follicle centre cell** (FCC) which belong to the B lymphocyte pathway: the **centroblast** which is a large, nucleated cell with a rapid rate of division, and the **centrocyte** which is a medium-sized cell with an irregular or 'cleaved' nucleus and a low mitotic rate. Neoplasms of the germinal centre are termed **centroblastic/centrocytic lymphomas** and in many cases recapitulate the architecture of the germinal centre and possess a follicular pattern. Less commonly centroblastic/centrocytic lymphomas may be partially or completely diffuse. Occasionally, tumours of germinal centres are composed exclusively of one cell type; either centrocytic or centroblastic. These lymphomas are always diffuse.

Malignancies of small lymphocytes are relatively common. They form a spectrum of disease ranging from cases with extensive marrow involvement, a peripheral blood lymphocytosis and inconspicuous lymphadenopathy to those whose clinical picture is dominated by lymph node involvement. The former picture is that of **chronic lymphocytic leukaemia** and the latter is termed **lymphocytic lymphoma**. The malignant cell appears identical in both processes and is a functionally immature B cell in the majority of cases. Lymphocytic lymphoma/B CLL is an indolent but incurable disease and many patients live for long periods, dying with the disease rather than as a direct result of it. A small percentage of lymphocytic lymphomas show evidence of early differentiation towards plasma cells. These are termed **lymphoplasmacytic lymphomas** and may be associated with the production of a monoclonal immunoglobulin. **Mycosis fungoides** is a cutaneous lymphocytic lymphoma which can spread to other organs and **Sézary's syndrome** is a related condition in which the skin changes are more diffuse and abnormal lymphocytes are found in the circulation. In both instances the abnormal cells are usually of T helper cell phenotype.

Lymphoblastic lymphomas are characterized by a proliferation of more primitive medium-sized, nucleolated cells. Lymphoblastic lymphomas can be categorized into three main types: T cell, B cell and null cell. Many null cell lymphoblastic lymphomas express CD10 and are derived from pre-B cells. Lymphoblastic lymphomas have a poor prognosis and frequently become leukaemic. **Burkitt's lymphoma** is an unusual B lymphoblastic lymphoma which causes massive tumours in and around the jaw. It occurs in young African children who have had chronic malaria in conjunction with EB virus infection and responds dramatically to chemotherapy. It is characterized by a translocation between chromosomes 8 and 14 which brings the *C-MYC* oncogene in close proximity to an immunoglobulin heavy chain gene permitting continuous expression of the former. Post-thymic T cell lymphomas are relatively uncommon in Europe (approximately 10 per cent of all NHL) but are common in Japan and the Caribbean where they are associated with infection by the retrovirus HTLV I. The spectrum of T cell neoplasms appears at least as complex as B cell lymphomas and they also have a high frequency of cutaneous infiltration and hypercalcaemia.

Non-Hodgkin's lymphoma is usually treated with radiotherapy if localized and with single or combination chemotherapy if the disease is more extensive or aggressive. Most patients with a low-grade follicular lymphoma do moderately well but the remainder respond poorly. Trials of intensive chemotherapy followed by transplantation with autologous bone marrow purged of lymphoma cells have produced more favourable results.

Angioimmunoblastic lymphadenopathy with dysproteinaemia (AILD)

This condition is characterized by generalized lymphadenopathy, hepatosplenomegaly, skin rashes, fever and a polyclonal increase in serum IgG (and often IgA and IgM). Lymphoblastoid cells may be present in peripheral blood. The diagnosis is made on the histological changes observed in lymphoid tissue, i.e. a mixed cellular infiltrate containing immunoblasts, lymphocytes, plasma cells, eosinophils and histiocytes, marked proliferation of small blood vessels and deposition of an amorphous acidophilic material between the infiltrating cells. Anecdotal reports suggest that this condition may be triggered by various drugs, e.g. phenytoin or penicillin, or other antigens. A variety of autoantibodies are present and there is usually a haemolytic anaemia with a T cell lymphopenia and anergy on delayed hypersensitivity testing. Some cases spontaneously remit or respond to steroid treatment but 5–10 per cent of patients develop an immunoblastic lymphoma. The cellular infiltrate and blood vessel proliferation are probably due to cytokine release from the abnormal cells which are usually of T cell origin.

Monoclonal gammopathies

This is a group of disorders in which evidence of monoclonal proliferation is readily obtained due to the fact that the abnormal cells derive from terminal stages of the B cell maturation pathway (Fig. 17.1) and secrete large quantities of a chemically homogeneous immunoglobulin product. In **macroglobulinaemia**, the abnormal cell is a **B lymphoblast** which is found in lymph nodes, spleen and marrow and the secreted product is of class **IgM**. In **myeloma**, the abnormal cells resemble **plasma cells** and produce lesions in marrow-containing bones without involvement of secondary lymphoid organs and the secreted immunoglobulins are of classes **IgG**, **IgA**, **IgD** or **IgE**. The organ distribution of the abnormal cells in macroglobulinaemia is in keeping with the presence of IgM-producing plasma cells in the medulla of lymph nodes and red pulp of the spleen but the localization to the bone marrow of monoclonal plasma cells producing immunoglobulins of other isotypes is more difficult to explain unless these are cells which differentiate directly from pre-B cells in bone marrow or represent cells that have switched from IgM production and seeded secondarily in bone marrow.

MACROGLOBULINAEMIA

Virtually all the symptoms of this condition are due to the presence of a **monoclonal IgM** of κ or λ type secreted by a population of cells infiltrating lymph nodes, spleen, liver and bone marrow which give the appearance of a slowly growing lymphoplasmacytoid lymphoma. The pentameric nature of secreted IgM (1 million daltons molecular weight) leads to symptoms of blood **hyperviscosity** when levels exceed 30 g litre^{-1} and causes circulatory problems in the retina, central nervous system and extremities. Interaction of monoclonal IgM with the surfaces of platelets, red cells and neutrophils may cause bleeding, anaemia and infection and in some cases the abnormal protein behaves as a **cryoglobulin**, giving rise to cold-induced peripheral vasospasm, i.e. **Raynaud's phenomenon**.

In contrast to myeloma, lytic bone lesions and the production of plentiful free light chains are not features of this condition and thus bone pain, hypercalcaemia and renal failure are rarely seen. In contrast, rare cases of monoclonal monomeric (7S) IgM usually have the clinical features of myeloma (Table 17.2). Macroglobulinaemia is usually treated with prednisolone and a cytotoxic agent and by plasmapheresis when hyperviscosity or cryoglobulinaemia is a problem.

MYELOMA

This is a malignant proliferation of plasma cells secreting a single immunoglobulin isotype of class **IgG, IgA, IgD, IgE** or **7S IgM** and

Table 17.2 Incidence of monoclonal isotypes in myeloma.

MONOCLONAL ISOTYPES IN MYELOMA	
IgG	55%
IgA	20%
IgM*	0.5%
IgD	1.5%
IgE	0.01%
Light chain only	20%

*This refers to monomeric 7S IgM. Monoclonal pentameric 19S IgM occurs in macroglobulinaemia.

containing light chains of κ or λ type. In about 20 per cent of cases the plasma cells secrete light chains in the absence of a heavy chain (Table 17.2). The abnormal plasma cells accumulate in bone marrow, replacing the normal marrow elements, and cause **bone pain** and, in some cases, pathological fracture (Table 17.3). Decalcification of the surrounding bone and **hypercalcaemia** are due to the release of osteoclast activating factors. These factors include IL-1, IL-6 and TNF but IL-6 is the most potent and also mediates the effects of the other two. Levels of C-reactive protein (see p. 158) are also raised and can be used to monitor disease activity.

Interleukin-6 is the major cytokine controlling the differentiation of plasmablast cells into mature plasma cells and is an important growth factor for myeloma cells *in vitro*. In myelomatosis, it originates from other bone marrow cells, e.g. myeloid cells and monocytes, rather than from the myeloma cells, although the latter may well induce it by releasing cytokines such as IL-1. Monoclonal antibodies to IL-6 inhibit myeloma cell proliferation but it is not possible to achieve this *in vivo* because the levels of IL-6 are usually too high. However, corticosteroids such as dexamethasone, oestrogens, and inhibitors of IL-1 and TNF also inhibit IL-6 and are currently under investigation for the treatment of myelomatosis. Interferon-γ may also have a role in inhibiting IL-6 induced proliferation.

There is an increased incidence of **infection** due to the development of secondary hypogammaglobulinaemia, neutropenia or interaction of the monoclonal immunoglobulin (if of isotypes IgG1 or IgG3) with phagocytic cells. Patients often show a bleeding tendency due to interaction of the myeloma protein with platelets or coagulation factors. **Hyperviscosity** of the blood is less likely with increased levels of monomeric immunoglobulins but occurs when these approach $100\,g$ litre^{-1} and is particularly marked with IgG3 proteins which have a spontaneous tendency to aggregate. Some myeloma proteins also behave as **cryoglobulins** (see p. 256), giving rise to cold sensitivity phenomena.

CLINICAL FEATURES OF MYELOMA

Anaemia	>90%
Bone lesions	80%
Infection	50%
Hypercalcaemia	45%
Renal failure	45%

Table 17.3 Clinical features of myeloma at presentation.

Plasma cells normally synthesize an excess of **light chains** compared to their level of heavy chain production. Large quantities of monoclonal free light chains are produced in myeloma and this material, being of small molecular weight, passes readily into the urine. This feature has become known as **Bence-Jones protein** after the author of its first description in 1847. These excessive amounts of light chain can, however, be toxic to renal tubules, and other factors, e.g. hypercalcaemia, hyperuricaemia, amyloidosis and dehydration, also contribute toward the development of **myeloma kidney**.

A compact band is usually present on zone electrophoresis of serum (see p. 78) but this can have causes other than a monoclonal gammopathy. Monoclonal immunoglobulins are identified by **immuno-electrophoresis** (see Figs 6.10 & 17.2) and a diagnosis of myeloma cannot be excluded until this has been performed on serum and urine. Some patients will only show a monoclonal immunoglobulin in serum whereas others with 'Bence-Jones only' myeloma will only show the presence of light chains in urine unless there is impaired filtration due to renal failure. In more severely affected cases the immunoglobulins belonging to other classes are reduced, probably related to marrow infiltration and suppression of normal plasma cells.

Abnormal plasma cells are usually apparent on conventional examination of a bone marrow sample obtained by aspiration or trephine biopsy. Most patients show radiological evidence of bone destruction. Examination of bone marrow cells by immunofluorescence (see p. 98) is also useful in confirming the diagnosis of a monoclonal proliferation and in identifying the isotype.

The treatment of myeloma has been unsatisfactory with only a modest increase in survival following courses of melphalan (a cytotoxic drug) and prednisolone. However, the more aggressive use of combination therapy (e.g. vincristine, doxorubicin and steroids followed by high-dose melphalan) has improved the outlook in recent trials and the application of bone marrow transplantation (allogeneic or autologous), interferon, and inhibitors of IL-6 offer further promise.

Benign monoclonal gammopathy

Monoclonal immunoglobulins also occur in other conditions (Table 17.4) and some patients have monoclonal proteins which are either transient or persistent but of undetermined significance and not associated with malignant disease. This condition has been called **benign monoclonal gammopathy** but the diagnosis is difficult to establish prospectively. However, patients who have a level of monoclonal immunoglobulin less

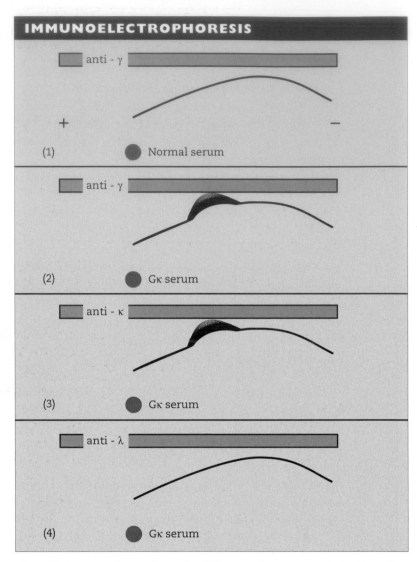

Fig. 17.2 Immunoelectrophoresis of (1) normal serum reacted with anti-γ and (2, 3 and 4) a serum containing an IgG κ monoclonal protein reacted with anti-γ, anti-κ and anti-λ respectively. Normal serum gives a long and heterogeneous line of IgG precipitation extending from close to the application well (shaded circle) to the cathodal end. The monoclonal IgG κ protein gives a restricted 'bow' of precipitation (with the anti-γ and anti-κ reagents) which deviates from the normal IgG line and extends upwards toward the horizontal trough in which the antiserum is placed. In myeloma and macroglobulinaemia, the amount of monoclonal protein may be so great that the precipitate redissolves in antigen excess (i.e. along its lower edge) and may merge with the antiserum trough. This can be overcome by examining the serum at greater dilution.

CAUSES OF MONOCLONAL GAMMOPATHY

Myeloma
Macroglobulinaemia
Non-Hodgkin's lymphoma
Chronic lymphocytic leukaemia
Primary cold agglutinin disease
Benign monoclonal gammopathy

Table 17.4 Causes of monoclonal gammopathy.

than 20 g l^{-1}, have few (< 5 per cent) plasma cells in bone marrow, do not show suppression of other immunoglobulin classes, do not have an excess of urinary light chains and lack bone lesions, show a much more benign course, and may remain well for many years. However, careful follow-up has revealed that about 20 per cent of such patients develop myeloma, macroglobulinaemia or amyloidosis within a 10-year period.

HEAVY CHAIN DISEASES

Rare patients have been identified who show excessive production of free heavy chains, e.g. the α chain of IgA, the γ chain of IgG, the μ chain of IgM or the δ chain of IgD. **Alpha chain disease** is the commonest of this group. It is associated with severe diarrhoea, malabsorption, abdominal pain and weight loss and is also called Immunoproliferative small-intestinal disease (IPSID). The small gut shows diffuse infiltration with lymphoplasmacytoid cells secreting α chain dimers which usually show deletion of the variable (V_H) region. Free α chains can be detected in serum by the technique of **immunoselection** in which the sample is electrophoresed through agarose-containing antisera reactive with κ and λ chains in order to precipitate all the intact immunoglobulin molecules, thus leaving any free heavy chains to react with an anti-α chain reagent in a second zone.

The incomplete nature of the abnormal immunoglobulin in this condition makes it difficult to be certain that this is a monoclonal abnormality. Some cases have remitted following oral treatment with antibiotics but most cases transform into an immunoblastic lymphoma of B cell type. Gamma chain disease behaves like a malignant lymphoma and γ chain fragments (often of the $\gamma3$ subclass) can be detected in serum. Mu chain disease resembles chronic lymphocytic leukaemia with pentameric μ chain fragments present in serum and κ light chains in the urine, suggesting a monoclonal proliferation. A case of δ chain disease resembled myeloma but with free δ chains in the serum.

Cryoglobulinaemia

The serum of some patients contains proteins which spontaneously precipitate or form gel-like polymers at temperatures below 37°C and are termed **cryoglobulins**. About 25 per cent of cases are **type I** due to the presence of **monoclonal** immunoglobulins which have an intrinsic tendency to cryoprecipitate (Table 17.5). **Type II** cryoglobulins are of mixed type (**monoclonal–polyclonal**) and contain a monoclonal protein (most often of class IgM) with rheumatoid factor-like activity, i.e. it has specificity for IgG and forms complexes with it. These also tend to precipitate in the cold. This type of cryoglobulinaemia is associated with various kinds of lymphoproliferative disease including macroglobulinaemia. Overall, approximately 10 per cent of monoclonal IgM proteins have cryoglobulin activity: half of them spontaneously (type I) and half as a complex with IgG (type II). Some of the latter give rise to a clinical picture consisting of purpura, arthralgia, lymphadenopathy and hepatosplenomegaly in the absence of other primary disease—a condition known as **mixed essential cryoglobulinaemia** (MEC).

The remaining 50 per cent of patients with cryoglobulinaemia (**type III**) are of mixed polyclonal type (**polyclonal–polyclonal**) in which polyclonal IgM rheumatoid factor-like antibodies complex with IgG and precipitate in the cold. These patients usually have an obvious immune

TYPES OF CRYOGLOBULINAEMIA

Type	Cases (%)	Composition	Serum level	Diseases
I	25	Monoclonal Ig IgM, IgG or IgA	$1–30\,g\,l^{-1}$	Macroglobulinaemia Myeloma Lymphoma
II	25	Monoclonal–polyclonal Ig IgM–IgG IgG–IgG IgA–IgG	$1–5\,g\,l^{-1}$	Macroglobulinaemia Lymphoma CLL* MEC†
III	50	Polyclonal–polyclonal Ig IgM–IgG	$0.1–1\,g\,l^{-1}$	Systemic lupus Sjögren's disease Rheumatoid arthritis Vasculitis Chronic infection

* CLL, Chronic lymphocytic leukaemia; † MEC, mixed essential cryoglobulinaemia.

Table 17.5 Types of cryoglobulinaemia.

complex disease, e.g. systemic lupus, rheumatoid arthritis, or chronic infection, e.g. bacterial endocarditis. In each case the symptoms can be alleviated by plasmapheresis and/or the use of prednisolone and cytotoxic agents, although treatment is directed against the primary disorder where possible.

Amyloidosis

Virchoff gave the term **amyloid** or 'starch-like' to the material that stains with iodine which he observed in tissue following chronic inflammation. These days this material is detected by the use of dyes such as Congo red or thioflavine t; by its birefringence under polarized light or by its fibrillary structure on electron microscopy. The amyloid fibrils which deposit in tissues are, in fact, all derived from protein precursors (Table 17.6) and are formed following enzymatic action which promotes their polymerization in β-conformation. Amyloid deposits also contain a non-fibrillary glycoprotein — amyloid P component — which is derived from a serum protein designated SAP.

Light chain-associated or lymphoproliferative amyloidosis occurs in several related conditions, including myeloma, and follows the excessive production of monoclonal free light chains. It can affect various tissues including the heart, kidneys and peripheral nerves, and is an important

AMYLOIDOSIS AND FIBRIL PROTEINS		
Clinical type	Amyloid protein	Precursor protein
Lymphoproliferative Myeloma Macroglobulinaemia Heavy chain disease Primary amyloidosis	Amino-terminal (variable region) of light chains (AL)	Light chains
Reactive systemic Chronic inflammation Chronic infection Malignant disease	Protein A (AA)	Serum amyloid A apolipoprotein (SAA)
Following chronic haemodialysis	β_2-microglobulin (Aβ_2M)	β_2-microglobulin (β_2M)
Heredofamilial amyloidosis	AA or prealbumen	SAA or prealbumen

Table 17.6 Types of amyloidosis and their fibril proteins.

cause of myeloma kidney (see p. 253). The main component of the amyloid fibrils is a protein, designated AL, which consists of light chains or fragments thereof which include the V_L domain. Another form of amyloid protein occurs in association with chronic stimulation of the immune system and is called amyloid A protein (AA). It has a circulating serum precursor (SAA) which is an acute phase protein (see p. 158). This reactive form of amyloidosis affects the liver, spleen and kidneys causing enlargement and functional impairment. β_2-microglobulin and pre-albumen are also able to form amyloid fibrils when their metabolism is disturbed as in chronic haemodialysis and various forms of familial amyloidosis, respectively.

KEY POINTS

1 Abnormal proliferation of the cells of the immune system takes many forms, e.g. leukaemia, lymphoma, myeloma, macroglobulinaemia and heavy chain diseases. Cryoglobulinaemia and amyloidosis are also associated with the abnormal production of proteins involved in the immune response.

2 The characterization of proteins present on the surface and in the cytoplasm of lymphocytes and myeloid cells is the chief means of diagnosing and identifying the abnormal cell in the six main types of acute leukaemia which vary in their management and prognosis.

3 Epstein–Barr virus is a potent stimulus for B cell proliferation, and infection with it usually results in the self-limiting condition – infectious mononucleosis. However, this virus is also implicated in the pathogenesis of Hodgkin's disease, non-Hodgkin's lymphoma and Burkitt's lymphoma and the development of these conditions is likely to be associated with as yet unidentified forms of genetic or acquired susceptibility.

The origin of the disease-defining cell in Hodgkin's disease – the Reed–Sternberg cell – is still debated but most of the evidence suggests a lymphoid source. More than 90 per cent of non-Hodgkin's lymphomas are derived from the B cell lineage.

4 The monoclonal gammopathies are caused by the uncontrolled proliferation of a single clone of plasma cells (in myelomatosis) or B lymphoblasts (in macroglobulinaemia). In macroglobulinaemia, the excess production of pentameric IgM is associated with hyperviscosity and cryoglobulinaemia. In myeloma, the monoclonal immunoglobulin can be of class IgG, IgA, IgD, IgE or monomeric IgM. Decalcification, hypercalcaemia and bone pain is mediated by cytokine release initiated by the abnormal plasma cells and agents that inhibit IL-6 are under investigation for the treatment of myelomatosis.

5 Amyloidosis is caused by the deposition of amyloid fibrils in body tissues. It arises when various kinds of proteins are over-produced in certain chronic diseases and polymerize following enzymatic action.

Further reading

Fossum S. & Ford W.L. (1985) The organisation of cell populations within lymph nodes: their origin, life history and functional relationships. *Histopathology*, **9**, 469–499.

Husby G. (1993) The acute phase response and the pathogenesis of reactive, amyloid A amyloidosis. In Lachmann P.J., Peters, D.K., Rosen F.S. & Walport M.J. eds, *Clinical Aspects of Immunology*, 5th edn. Blackwell Scientific Publications, Oxford.

Klein B., Zhang X.-G., Lu Z.-Y. & Bataille R. (1995) Interleukin-6 in human multiple myeloma. *Blood*, **85**, 863–872.

Kyle R.A. (1991) Plasma cell proliferative diseases. In Hoffman R., Banz E.J., Shattil S.J., Furie B. & Cohen H.J. eds, *Haematology: Basic Principles and Practice*. Churchill Livingstone, London.

Leibowitz D. (1995) Epstein–Barr virus – an old dog with new tricks. *New England Journal of Medicine*, **332**, 55–57.

Malpas J.S., Bergsagel D.E. & Kyle R.A. (1995) *Myeloma*. Oxford University Press, Oxford.

Matutes E. (1995) Contribution of immunophenotype in the diagnosis and classification of haemopoietic malignancies. *Journal of Clinical Pathology*, **48**, 194–197.

Rabbits T.H. (1991) Translocation, master genes, and differences between the origin of acute and chronic leukemias. *Cell*, **67**, 641–644.

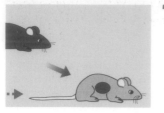

CHAPTER 18

Transplantation

Histocompatibility systems

Vertebrates possess the ability to reject most cells or tissues obtained from sources other than those of their own genetic type and some invertebrates also display incompatibility reactions, e.g. genetically distinct corals growing on a reef. The speed and vigour with which tissues are rejected are related to their mutual degree of foreignness and the terms used to describe these differences are summarized in Fig. 18.1. Most of these inherited chemical differences belong to the **major histocompatibility complex** (MHC) designated **H2** in the mouse and **HLA** in man and are described in more detail in Chapter 2. Other minor systems have a weaker influence on tissue compatibility. The genes of the MHC code for two kinds of cell surface glycoprotein: **class I** are present on all nucleated cells whereas **class II** glycoproteins are normally only present on cells involved in immune recognition, e.g. antigen presenting cells, B cells and T helper cells (see p. 31).

It has been estimated that at least 10 per cent of peripheral T cells can express reactivity to alloantigens. This seemingly inappropriate ability to react to foreign tissue specificities does, however, have important physiological significance — implicit in the phenomenon of **dual recognition** (see p. 29 and Figs 2.8 & 4.5).

In essence, T lymphocytes — unlike B lymphocytes — recognize antigenic determinants conjointly with self HLA glycoproteins. T helper cells recognize antigen in association with class II glycoprotein on the surface of specialized antigen presenting cells whereas cytotoxic T cells recognize antigen in association with class I glycoprotein on the surface of any nucleated cell. This ensures that each subpopulation of T lymphocytes is guided to react with antigen in a functionally relevant situation.

TERMS FOR FOREIGNNESS OF TISSUES			
RELATIONSHIP	NOUNS	ADJECTIVES	
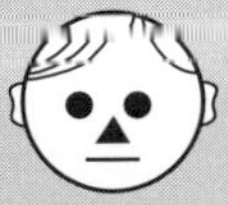	Autograft	Syngeneic	Autologous
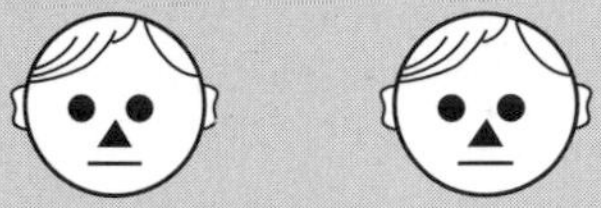	Isograft	Syngeneic	Isologous
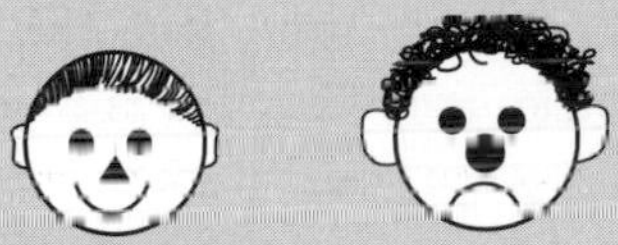	Allograft	Allogeneic	Homologous
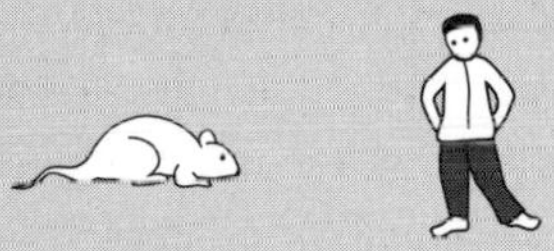	Xenograft	Xenogeneic	Heterologous

Fig. 18.1 Terms used to describe immunological relationships.

Recent studies with T cells specific for peptide antigens have demonstrated that such cells often show preferential binding for certain *allogeneic* histocompatibility glycoproteins, reinforcing the view that T cells see foreign tissues as 'self + x' (see p. 44).

The rejection process

The specificity and tempo of allograft rejection has already been illustrated in Fig. 1.2. Skin allografts continue to look normal for about 5 days after grafting but perivascular infiltration with lymphocytes develops around day 7, followed by vascular obstruction and leakage with oedema and necrosis of the graft epithelium. Necrosis is usually complete by day 14 when the graft takes on a black and shrunken appearance. This process is accelerated if the recipient's lymphocytes have direct vascular access to the graft, e.g. as in a renal transplant.

AFFERENT LIMB

For grafts which do not involve the construction of a vascular anastomosis, the process of recognition or 'sensitization' usually requires intact lymphatic access, and grafts placed in specially constructed skin flaps or epithelial pouches or within the central nervous system may avoid rejection indefinitely: these locations have been referred to as **privileged sites**. The critical stimulus for the rejection of human tissues placed in unprivileged locations is the expression of class II HLA glycoproteins on the surface of antigen presenting cells (Fig. 18.2). The T helper cell recognizes foreign determinants in association with class II glycoproteins and allogeneic HLA glycoproteins are recognized as a form of modified 'self'. Class I differences alone may not be sufficient to *induce* an allograft response. The necessity for class II differences to be present and that these should be expressed on intact cells is illustrated by the use of **mixed lymphocyte culture** (MLC) as an *in vitro* correlate of the afferent limb of the allograft response (Fig. 18.3). MLC relies on the ability of mixtures of mononuclear cells from non-identical individuals to stimulate each other in culture even when identical at HLA-A and HLA-B loci and this led to the identification of the HLA-D class II locus. Variations at class II loci are now more usually characterized by serology or DNA typing.

A major advance in recent years has been the realization that much of the immunogenicity of grafted tissues is due to the presence of donor antigen presenting cells—originally referred to as **passenger leucocytes** but now often called **dendritic cells**—which bear allogeneic class II molecules and present them directly to the recipient T helper cell without a requirement for intracellular processing (Fig. 18.2). Very few of these dendritic cells are required to elicit an allograft response and if they are removed prior to grafting so that induction of the allograft response has to occur via processing by recipient antigen presenting cells then the response is very much weaker and less immunosuppressive therapy is required to prevent rejection. Only occasional processed fragments will resemble allogeneic class II and this route of sensitization is very much less efficient than the direct presentation of allogeneic class II molecules by donor dendritic cells to which the T helper cells can respond directly. The relative immunogenicity of different allogeneic tissues follows the

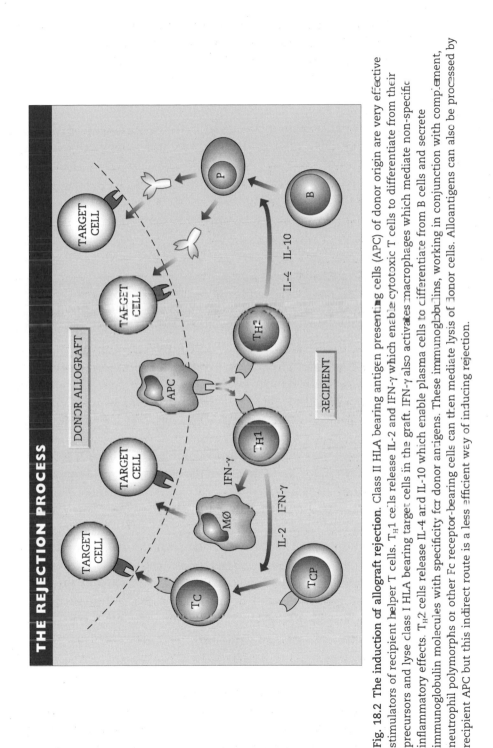

Fig. 18.2 The induction of allograft rejection. Class II HLA bearing antigen presenting cells (APC) of donor origin are very effective stimulators of recipient helper T cells. T_H1 cells release IL-2 and IFN-γ which enable cytotoxic T cells to differentiate from their precursors and lyse class I HLA bearing target cells in the graft. IFN-γ also activates macrophages which mediate non-specific inflammatory effects. T_H2 cells release IL-4 and IL-10 which enable plasma cells to differentiate from B cells and secrete immunoglobulin molecules with specificity for donor antigens. These immunoglobulins, working in conjunction with complement, neutrophil polymorphs or other Fc receptor-bearing cells can then mediate lysis of donor cells. Alloantigens can also be processed by recipient APC but this indirect route is a less efficient way of inducing rejection.

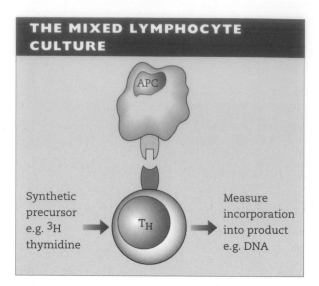

Fig. 18.3 The mixed lymphocyte culture (MLC). When allogeneic mononuclear cells purified from peripheral blood are set up in culture with mononuclear cells of self origin, the class II-bearing cells act as antigen presenting cells (APC) and activate a proportion of the T helper cell population, i.e. the MLC mirrors the initial steps of allograft rejection as depicted in Fig. 18.2. This is quantified by adding a radio-labelled precursor of DNA, RNA or protein which becomes incorporated into these products as the cells increase synthesis and proceed to cell division.

descending sequence of bone marrow, skin, pancreatic islets, gut, heart, kidney and liver, and largely relates to the quantity of class II-bearing cells within them.

EFFERENT LIMB

Once T helper cells become activated then the normal cooperative events (including the release of interleukins) enable cytotoxic T cells to differentiate from cytotoxic precursors (T_{CP}) with specificity for class I-bearing allogeneic cells, and B cells to differentiate into plasma cells secreting antibody of allogeneic specificity. Graft rejection is also associated with the activation of macrophages which are induced by interferon (IFN)-γ.

The response to an allograft transferred a second time—the 'second set' reaction—is more vigorous due to an expanded population of effector T cells which can operate without T helper cell stimulation. Specific antibody may also contribute to the more rapid rejection process. The balance between T cell and antibody-mediated effects varies according to the circumstance, e.g. the **acute rejection** of renal allografts is predominantly T cell-mediated whereas **chronic rejection** can be due to either, or to a combination of both. In contrast, the dramatic events of **hyperacute rejection**, in which the kidney develops vascular stasis with platelet aggregation, neutrophil adherence and loss of function, are due to the presence of complement-fixing antibody in the recipient's circulation. This is usually avoided by a pretransplant cross-matching procedure in which the recipient's serum is examined for the presence of antibody cytotoxic to donor cells.

Ways of modifying the rejection process

Patients afflicted with end-stage organ failure are terminally ill or severely disabled, and when the kidneys are involved, face the prospect of regular dialysis for the rest of their lives. The realization that patients in this category can be restored to a healthy and useful life following organ transplantation has given enormous momentum to the search for ways of ameliorating the normal allograft response (Table 18.1).

HLA TYPING AND MATCHING

Typing of kidney donors and their recipients at the major class I loci — **HLA-A** and **HLA-B**—demonstrated that the degree of mismatch affected graft survival although the extreme polymorphism of these two loci means that it is relatively unusual to obtain a complete match between the four possible specificities of both donor and recipient. Incompatibility at the HLA-C locus seems to have little effect on graft survival. The introduction of **HLA-DR** typing by serological means indicated that matching for the rather smaller number of specificities at this class II locus had an even greater effect on graft survival in keeping with the pre-eminent role of class II glycoproteins in invoking the allograft response. However, the deleterious effect of mismatched grafts has

FACTORS PROMOTING GRAFT SURVIVAL
HLA typing and matching
Source and preparation of the graft
Selection and preparation of the recipient
Monitoring the allograft response
Non-specific immunosuppression
Specific immunosuppression (including the blood transfusion effect)

Table 18.1 Factors which promote graft survival.

diminished following the addition of cyclosporin to modern immunosuppressive regimens and the urgent need of individual patients and the difficulties of finding perfect matches means that mismatched grafts are often used in renal transplantation. This is less feasible in bone marrow transplantation where the requirements are more stringent (see below).

The procedures by which the limited supply of cadaveric organs is matched to the recipients' characteristics has reached an advanced state of organization in many countries through national and international transplant agencies.

SOURCE AND PREPARATION OF THE GRAFT

Most renal allografts are obtained from unrelated cadaveric donors and are often transported considerable distances in order to provide a satisfactory match between donor and recipient. The period of time during which the kidney is not perfused with an oxygenated blood supply (ischaemia time) is critical and should not exceed 45 minutes at 37°C or 24 hours at 4°C. For liver transplantation the cold ischaemia time is reduced to about 8 hours.

Living related donors are sometimes used in renal transplantation and in this situation it is possible to match entire haplotypes (see Fig. 16.2, p. 237). Living donors are the normal source of bone marrow for transplantation and can donate on successive occasions.

The pretreatment of grafts with antibodies specific for class II-bearing dendritic cells linked to cytotoxic agents may render the graft considerably less immunogenic. Purging of bone marrow to remove T lymphocytes is now widely used as a means of reducing the incidence and severity of graft-versus-host disease and is discussed further on p. 273.

SELECTION AND PREPARATION OF THE RECIPIENT

Many patients awaiting renal transplantation develop cytotoxic antibodies reactive with lymphocytes or endothelium following previous transfusion, grafting, pregnancy or infection. This state of presensitization to allogeneic tissue can lead to hyperacute rejection of a renal allograft and it is now routine procedure to perform a cytotoxic cross-match between the recipient's serum and the donor's lymphocytes. However, only antibodies with HLA-A and HLA-B specificity cause hyperacute rejection. Antibodies reactive with products of class II loci are much less damaging and other autoreactive antibodies may even facilitate graft survival. Soon after renal transplantation began it was noticed that the strict avoidance of blood transfusion to prevent presensitization *increased* the chances of graft rejection and a protocol of pregraft exposure to allogeneic blood was introduced in most renal transplant centres (see p. 271).

MONITORING THE ALLOGRAFT RESPONSE

Allograft rejection conjures up a dramatic picture of immunological events which should be eminently suitable to monitoring by the examination of peripheral blood for changes in antibody or lymphocyte characteristics. Many attempts, involving a wide range of antibody and lymphocyte assays, have failed to provide a clinically useful means of distinguishing rejection episodes from other events such as infection, or one that gives sufficient warning to be able to modify the outcome by therapeutic intervention. This is due to the fact that the specific cells and antibodies of interest are mostly preoccupied within the graft and thus not available for peripheral sampling.

The introduction of **fine needle aspiration biopsy** of cells within renal grafts has been a major advance. Samples (10 μl) can be removed on alternate days without significant damage to the graft. The nature of the cellular infiltrate is a useful guide to the development of rejection and its severity: the presence of T and B cell blasts occurs early in the rejection process and infiltration with monocytes indicates severe and possibly irreversible change. A significant improvement in the survival of cardiac allografts—for which HLA matching is not attempted—followed the introduction of serial myocardial biopsy in order to observe the early histological changes of rejection. Otherwise, one is left with the non-immunological observation of graft function, using physical, biochemical, isotopic or electrocardiographic techniques and these changes can be very non-specific.

NON-SPECIFIC IMMUNOSUPPRESSION

The potency of the antiallograft response is such that none of the factors cited thus far is sufficient to achieve graft survival without the administration of drugs which suppress the immune system non-specifically. It is only following the exchange of grafts between identical twins (i.e. isografts) or when transferring tissue within the same individual (i.e. autografts) that immunosuppressive measures are unnecessary. In allotransplantation most rejection episodes occur during the first 3 months but a reduced level of immunosuppressive treatment is required indefinitely in most cases.

In the early days of renal transplantation, immunosuppression was usually achieved using the antiproliferative drug, **azathioprine** (in a dose of c. 2.5 mg kg^{-1} day^{-1}), in conjunction with the powerful anti-inflammatory corticosteroid, **prednisolone**, (initially in a dose of 30–100 mg day^{-1} and gradually reduced toward a maintenance dose of 10 mg day^{-1}). The introduction of **cyclosporin**—a fungal metabolite—in the early 1980s had a major impact on graft survival and the combination of low-dose cyclosporin with azathioprine and prednisolone is now used in many centres.

Azathioprine inhibits DNA and RNA synthesis and blocks IL-2 production by lymphocytes. It can cause bone marrow aplasia and frequent monitoring of the white cell count is required. Corticosteroids probably have an effect on T cell function in addition to their anti-inflammatory effect. They have many side-effects (Table 18.2) but these are less of a

SIDE-EFFECTS OF IMMUNOSUPPRESSION

Infection
Viral, e.g. CMV, HSV, varicella-zoster virus
Fungal, e.g. *Aspergillus, Candida, Pneumocystis*
Bacterial, e.g. tuberculosis, *Listeria, Nocardia*

Malignancy
Lymphomas
Skin tumours

Antiproliferative effects
Marrow suppression   Infertility*
Ulceration of GI tract   Hair loss*
                             Cystitis*

Teratogenesis

Steroid effects
Cushingoid appearance   Osteoporosis
Hypertension   Avascular bone necrosis
Diabetes   Cataracts
Peptic ulceration   Myopathy
Stunted growth

Cyclosporin
Nephrotoxicity   Hypercholesterolaemia
Hirsutism   Hypertension
Gum hypertrophy   Hepatotoxicity

Antilymphocyte globulin
Serum sickness, fever

* Seen particularly with cyclophosphamide.

Table 18.2 Side-effects of non-specific immunosuppression.

problem with the smaller dosage used in modern triple therapy. Cyclosporin binds to a calcium-dependent intracellular protein, cyclophilin, and inhibits the production of IL-2 by helper T cells. It does, however, have several important side-effects including nephrotoxicity, hirsutism, gum hypertrophy, hypercholesterolaemia, hypertension and hepatotoxicity, most of which are dose-related.

Several other immunosuppressive drugs are under evaluation, e.g. tacrolimus (FK 506), sirolimus (rapamycin), and mofetil (an antimetabolite). Tacrolimus resembles cyclosporin in its effect on the proteins involved in IL-2 production although its chemical structure is very different. It has similar side-effects to cyclosporin with the exception of hirsutism and gum hypertrophy. Sirolimus resembles tacrolimus in structure but acts distal to IL-2 production.

Antilymphocyte or **antithymocyte globulin** has been in use for many years but lacks a standardized bioassay to quantify its potency and preparations raised in other species can induce serum sickness. It is mostly used to treat acute rejection episodes that have failed to respond to a high dose of corticosteroid. Various monoclonal antibodies to lymphocyte surface proteins have been evaluated, e.g. anti-CD3, anti-CD4 and anti-CD8, and molecular techniques have been developed to incorporate their hypervariable regions into immunoglobulin molecules of human sequence (a technique known as 'reshaping'). However, serious infection has been a problem in some patients treated with these preparations and this emphasizes the overall limitation of non-specific immunosuppression. Antibodies reactive with the IL-2 receptor are also being investigated and may prove less devastating to the immune system.

Opportunistic infection is still a major cause of death in most transplantation programmes and emphasizes the need for more sophisticated forms of immunosuppression. The small but significant increase in the incidence of lymphomas and skin tumours is almost certainly due to impaired immunity to oncogenic viruses. The subject of secondary immunodeficiency is discussed in more detail in Chapter 13.

SPECIFIC IMMUNOSUPPRESSION

The prospect of inducing antigen-specific immunosuppression at will in the adult animal has been the goal of transplantation immunology since the 1950s when Medawar and his colleagues were able to induce a similar state in neonatal mice (Fig. 18.4). Experiment 1 demonstrates the normal rejection of a strain A skin graft by a mouse of the allogeneic B strain. Experiment 2 shows that if cells from strain A mice are inoculated into newborn mice of strain B then the latter animals accept skin grafts derived from strain A throughout their adult life having become specifi-

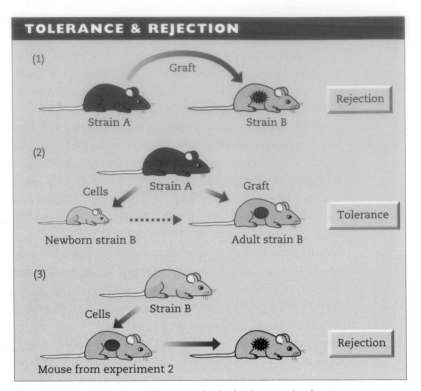

TOLERANCE & REJECTION

(1) Strain A — Graft → Strain B — Rejection

(2) Strain A — Cells → Newborn strain B ⋯⋯▶ Adult strain B — Graft → Tolerance

(3) Strain B — Cells → Mouse from experiment 2 → Rejection

Fig. 18.4 The induction of **immunological tolerance** in the mouse. Normally, skin grafts from strain A are rejected by the allogeneic strain B (experiment 1). However, if an animal of strain B is injected with cells from strain A when newborn it becomes tolerant to skin grafts from strain A for the rest of its life (experiment 2). This state of immunological tolerance can be broken by transferring lymphocytes from a strain B animal (that has not been pretreated) to a tolerant mouse. This is followed by prompt rejection of the strain A graft (experiment 3). These experiments were first performed by Billingham, Brent and Medawar (1956, *Nature*, **172**, 603–606).

cally tolerant of this histocompatibility type. That the tolerant animals are immunologically normal apart from their specific unresponsiveness to allografts from strain A is demonstrated in experiment 3 in which the natural tendency to reject the strain A graft the animal already bears is restored by the infusion of cells from a strain B animal that has not been pretreated with strain A cells when newborn. This kind of immunological tolerance is attainable in the mouse because of its immunological immaturity at birth and does not apply to most other mammals, including man.

Many other attempts have been made to induce **immunological tolerance** in adult animals and often with considerable success but the means by which graft acceptance has been achieved have not usually been clinically applicable or acceptable. It has been known for many years that the administration of graft-specific antibody can promote graft accept- ance although there is always a risk of hyperacute rejection. This phenomenon of antibody-mediated **enhancement** has been studied extensively and, at one stage, received limited clinical application for renal transplantation. In experiments where prolonged graft acceptance has been achieved by this means it is clear that the initial phase of induction (or passive enhancement) achieved by antibody is replaced by a mainten- ance phase (of active enhancement) in which other mechanisms operate. Enhancement can also be actively induced by the administration of allogeneic cells or cell extracts prior to transplantation. These effects have usually been achieved across relatively minor transplantation bar- riers and only succeed in some donor–recipient combinations. When successful, the animals bearing enhanced grafts tend to show a pro- gressive unresponsiveness to the donor strain. Some clinical examples have been recorded in which graft recipients have gradually 'adapted' to their allografts and been able to have most or all of their immunosuppressive drugs withdrawn.

Experimental studies have shown that the initial antibody-mediated phase of enhancement consists of the depletion of allogeneic class II- bearing cells from the graft. This may be achieved by a direct cytotoxic effect or may involve opsonization by phagocytic cells. Other experimen- tal models support the proposal that the maintenance phase of enhance- ment is due to the progressive development of **T suppressor cells**. A third explanation concerns the development of **auto-anti-idiotype antibodies** (idiotypes and anti-idiotypes are described on p. 82). Exper- imentally, it has been possible to demonstrate that the injection of T lymphocytes bearing idiotypes specific for allogeneic specificities can induce anti-idiotype antibodies which will suppress allograft responses. However, it is usually necessary to inject idiotype-bearing cells or mol- ecules in the presence of powerful adjuvants — a procedure which is not applicable to clinical transplantation. It is possible that suppressor cells which act to enhance graft acceptance may achieve this by expressing anti idiotype activity (see below).

THE BLOOD TRANSFUSION EFFECT

The realization that blood transfusion prior to allografting paradoxically increased graft survival led to the inclusion of this procedure in renal transplantation programmes. The efficacy of donor-specific transfusions in living related kidney transplantation could well be due to a specific effect akin to tolerance or enhancement. The fact that single random transfusions had a beneficial effect in around 25 per cent of patients receiving unrelated cadaveric grafts was more difficult to explain although the appearance of suppressor cells with anti-idiotype specificity has been documented in animal models. Minor histocompatibility determinants may be important in the transfusion effect which may follow the release of specific or non-specific factors from suppressor cells induced by transfusion. However, the magnitude of the transfusion effect has waned following the introduction of cyclosporin and many centres have abandoned the policy of pretransplant transfusion.

RECURRENT AND TRANSFERRED DISEASE

Quite a few diseases leading to end-stage organ failure have an immunological pathogenesis and in these (as well as other conditions) it is possible that the original disease will recur in the transplanted organ. This problem is well documented in renal transplantation and the frequency of recurrence in dense deposit disease and focal glomerulosclerosis negates the value of transplantation. IgA nephropathy, Goodpasture's disease and Henoch–Schonlein purpura also recur but with less severity.

The transplantation of pancreatic islets is under investigation as a means of reversing type I (insulin-dependent) diabetes. However, specific destruction of the insulin-producing β cells can occur soon after allografting, emphasizing the role of the immune system in this disease. Cardiac allografts often fail because of atherosclerosis, which may resemble the patient's original disease, and individuals who receive a graft for congestive cardiomyopathy are prone to develop a lymphoma. It is not unusual for leukaemia to recur in some patients treated with bone marrow transplantation (BMT) but, rarely, the cells of the recurrent leukaemia have been shown to be of donor origin, suggesting transfection of an oncogene (see Chapter 17). Several examples of the transfer of atopic or autoimmune disease by BMT have also been recorded.

The transfer of infection and malignancy are other possible hazards of organ grafting. In one case, a carcinoma developed following transfer of a kidney from a donor who was later found to have malignant disease. Fortunately, the tumour was rejected with the graft when immunosuppressive therapy was terminated.

Bone marrow transplantation

An advantage of bone marrow transplantation is that live donors are used and can be sources of marrow on successive occasions. A problem which is almost unique to BMT is that allograft reactions can occur in both directions, i.e. **graft-versus-host** (GVH) and **host-versus-graft** (HVG). This means that tissue matching has to be closer than is required for organ transplantation and involves mixed lymphocyte culture as well as serological or DNA typing at class I and class II loci. The permutations of the polymorphisms at these various loci are such that it is very unusual to find a satisfactory match from an unrelated donor and most marrow grafts are performed between siblings or parents and their offspring. The ideal situation, of course, is to have an identical twin. Marrow is aspirated from the iliac crests under local or general anaesthetic and is administered intravenously after passage through a wire mesh filter. The usual dose is c. 10^8 marrow cells kg^{-1} body weight.

Graft acceptance is achieved by giving **conditioning treatment** to the recipient. This usually takes the form of cyclophosphamide with total body irradiation; total lymphoid irradiation; antilymphocyte or antithymocyte globulin given in addition. The risks of intensive irradiation are considered unacceptable in children, who usually receive a course of busulphan. This treatment means that the recipient shows severe deficiency of all blood cells (pancytopenia) for 2–4 weeks until engraftment takes place. Intensive support is required during this period in the form of red cell, white cell and platelet transfusions, intravenous feeding, antibacterial agents and a protected pathogen-free environment. The immune responsiveness of the recipient is severely depleted during the first few months and infection is a considerable hazard. Interstitial pneumonia due to *Pneumocystis carinii* or cytomegalovirus is a common problem and varicella/zoster virus infections also occur.

GRAFT-VERSUS-HOST (GVH) DISEASE

This complication might be expected to occur in all bone marrow transfers that are not syngeneic but is only obvious in 35–45 per cent of cases although it seriously affects the outcome. It is characterized by a diffuse rash, fever, abdominal pain and diarrhoea with disturbed liver function and, almost always, superadded infection. Its incidence is proportional to the degree of mismatch between donor and recipient and in recent years it has become customary to pretreat the donor marrow with T cell-specific reagents in order to reduce the risk of GVH; a technique known as **purging** or **laundering**. Clearly, it is important to spare stem cells although how the subsequent differentiation of recipient-specific T cells from them is regulated is not clear. Possibly, such cells are brought under control by processes which survive the conditioning regimen and are comparable to the way in which T cell differentiation normally occurs in the thymus.

The introduction of cyclosporin A in the management of BMT has further reduced the incidence of GVH due to its preferential effect on helper T cells. However, in recent years it has become clear that there is a reciprocal relationship between the development of GVH and HVG responses in that a lower frequency of GVH associates with a higher incidence of graft rejection. The persisting problem of bone marrow graft rejection has led to trials of monoclonal antibodies specific for T cell subsets given to the recipients and this has increased the incidence of engraftment, e.g. when reagents specific for both CD4 and CD8 cells are combined. There is also evidence to suggest that the responsiveness of T cells within the graft may be beneficial in patients who receive BMT for leukaemia, i.e. an antileukaemia effect, although the existence of leukaemia-specific antigens is still a matter of debate.

INDICATIONS FOR BMT

The indications for BMT are the major immunodeficiencies, storage diseases and other inborn errors of metabolism, marrow aplasia and leukaemia (Table 18.3). BMT can be very successful in immunodeficiency and aplasia and the use of BMT to provide enzyme replacement for inborn errors is showing some promising results. BMT has given encouraging results in patients with acute myeloid leukaemia (AML) in their first remission, for without such intervention most patients die from their leukaemia. However, the success rate with chemotherapy for acute lymphoblastic leukaemia (ALL) is so much better that BMT is usually retained for a subsequent relapse although patients who are prone to relapse can be identified and offered BMT early on. BMT is receiving increasing application in chronic myeloid leukaemia (CML) where elective intervention during the chronic phase is favoured before progression to blast crisis and this often produces cytogenetic remission with disappearance of the Philadelphia chromosome (see p. 247).

AUTOLOGOUS TRANSPLANTATION

Some centres are adopting a more aggressive approach to certain haematological and solid tumours, in which the patient's marrow is stored before the patient is treated with intensive irradiation and/or chemotherapy, after which their marrow is returned. This also creates the opportunity to treat the marrow with antitumour antibodies and this approach has given encouraging results in ALL. A more recent development is **peripheral stem cell transfusion** in which stem cells are harvested from peripheral blood during the recovery phase of chemotherapy-induced neutropenia. The inclusion of granulocyte colony stimulating factor (G-CSF) in the regimen enhances the yield of stem cells

INDICATIONS FOR BMT

Immunodeficiency
Severe combined immunodeficiency (SCID)
Chronic granulomatous disease (CGD)
Leucocyte adhesion deficiency (LAD)
Wiskott–Aldrich syndrome

Storage/metabolic defects
Mucopolysaccharidoses, e.g. Hurler's disease
Lipidoses, e.g. Gaucher's disease

Marrow deficiency
Aplasia
Agranulocytosis

Leukaemia
Acute myeloid
Chronic myeloid
Acute lymphoblastic

Lymphoma
Hodgkin's disease
Non-Hodgkin's lymphoma

Myelomatosis

Haemoglobinopathies
Sickle-cell anaemia
Thalassaemia

Osteopetrosis

Table 18.3 Indications for bone marrow transplantation.

and the infusion of stem cells from peripheral blood as opposed to bone marrow reduces the hazard of contamination with malignant cells. This form of stem cell replacement may also be useful for allogeneic transplants although the normal donor would also need to be given G-CSF,

KEY POINTS

1 The critical stimulus for the rejection of foreign grafts is the recognition of class II HLA glycoproteins on the surface of allogeneic antigen presenting cells (APC) by helper T cells. Recipient APC can also process and present allogeneic class I HLA proteins but this indirect route of sensitization is less effective.

Continued on p. 276

KEY POINTS

2 Rejection is mediated primarily by cytotoxic T cells specific for allogeneic class I HLA proteins on graft cells. These cells differentiate from cytotoxic precursors under the influence of IL-2 released by T_H1 cells. Macrophages are activated by IFN-γ and plasma cells differentiate from B cells under the influence of IL-4 and IL-10. Both of these processes can augment destruction of the graft.

3 Graft survival can be promoted by:
  (a) close matching of HLA types between donor and recipient
  (b) ensuring that the donor tissue is optimally prepared
  (c) treating the recipient with an optimal immunosuppressive regimen
  (d) prompt detection and management of rejection episodes

4 All forms of non-specific immunosuppression have side-effects – some of which are serious – and it is hoped that a readily applicable form of antigen-specific immunosuppression will soon be available for clinical use.

5 The requirements for successful bone marrow transplantation (BMT) are even more stringent as incompatibility can be manifest as host-versus-graft or graft-versus-host reactions. BMT has been successfully used to correct various forms of immunodeficiency and metabolic defect and is being increasingly applied to the management of leukaemia, lymphoma, myelomatosis, haemoglobinopathies and marrow failure.

Further reading

Calne R.Y. (1994) Immunosuppression in liver transplantation. *New England Journal of Medicine*, **331**, 1154–1155.

Demirer T. & Bensinger W.I. (1995) Optimization of peripheral blood stem cell collections. *Current Opinion in Haematology*, **2**, 219–226.

Lechler R.I. & Wood K.J. (1993) The allograft response. In Lachman P.J., Peters D.K., Rosen F.S. & Walport M.J. eds, *Clinical Aspects of Immunology*, 5th edn. Blackwell Scientific Publications, Oxford.

Morris P.J. (1993) Kidney transplantation. In Lachman P.J., Peters D.K., Rosen F.S. & Walport M.J. eds, *Clinical Aspects of Immunology*, 5th edn. Blackwell Scientific Publications, Oxford.

Williams S.F. ed. (1993) Autologous bone marrow transplantation. *Haematology/Oncology Clinics of North America*, **7**(3).

Index